Dr. Eno's Guide to Living Powerfully with Diabetes

Eno Nsima-Obot, M.D.

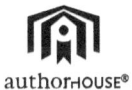

authorHOUSE®

AuthorHouse™
1663 Liberty Drive
Bloomington, IN 47403
www.authorhouse.com
Phone: 1-800-839-8640

First published by AuthorHouse 11/14/2011

ISBN: 978-1-4567-3538-8 (e)
ISBN: 978-1-4567-3539-5 (hc)
ISBN: 978-1-4567-3540-1 (sc)

Library of Congress Control Number: 2011901662

Printed in the United States of America

Dedication

This book is dedicated to the memory of Dorothy Allen Hill, my mother-in-law who died of complications related to diabetes in March 2008 at the tender age of eighty-two.

To my husband, George C. Hill—from the moment that you came into my life, you have been the wind beneath my wings. You helped me believe that I could conquer the world if I chose to. Thank you for your unfailing support. I love you, babe.

To my parents, Chief Eyo Udo Akpan and Bernice Akpan; to my sisters and brothers, Mfon Akpan, Victoria Akpan, Chris Akpan, and Spencer Akpan, who have watched in awe (and at times trepidation) as I searched for how I might live my purpose and be of service to mankind. I finally figured it out! This one is for you all. Thank you!

To my daughter, Emem Nsima Obot. I hope that as you grow up you realize the importance of living a life and leaving a legacy. Always reach for the stars. On mother's shoulders you can stand. I will love you forever.

To my patients of both the past and present—thank you for being there for me so that I could learn what it takes to truly be a partner in your care.

Contents

Foreword

During my years in practice as a primary care physician, I discovered that a lot of patients who had recently been diagnosed or who had been living with diabetes for quite some time had a lot of questions about their disease and did not have the resources sufficient to truly "get it."

With the number of people with diabetes expected to double to forty-four million in the next twenty-five years in the United States, we need to become more aware of measures to prevent or treat early diabetes now more than ever.

In my experience, a typical fifteen minute office visit is not enough time to answer all the questions or arm patients with the knowledge needed to move them forward. As the saying goes, "knowledge is power."

Spending time with patients and educating them about their disease process improves a patient's willingness to become fully engaged in their medical treatment, and in the long run, this has been found to yield better outcomes.

Research shows that patients do not understand up to 50 percent of the information that they are given during an encounter with a health-care provider, especially when that provider is a physician. It is my intention to provide individuals with knowledge of diabetes in an easy-to-understand format in order to help them live healthy and productive lives with diabetes.

I have written with simple yet illustrative phrases. In the book, I have set out to explain the different aspects of diabetes care, using each letter of the alphabet.

I have also created a space for journaling and reflection on what each aspect of care means to you and the steps that you will need to take to make a difference in living with diabetes.

By empowering people with knowledge, they are able to make better informed and healthier decisions.

This manual has been a long time coming, and it is for all my patients who have heard me mutter, "I have a book in my head and I just need to get it down on paper." Here it is! This book is for you all.

In addition to being a physician, I am also trained as a life coach. In this manual, my goal is to focus more on wellness than disease. My assertion is that being diagnosed with diabetes does not mean that you cannot live a life that focuses on being healthy and doing things to support your well-being. In fact, it is a call to embrace a wellness lifestyle with enthusiasm and an optimistic attitude.

There are several ways that this manual can be used. It can be used as a personal manual. Express your thoughts and feelings in the journal entries.

It could also be used as a manual for group classes during which members could meet on a weekly basis and address each aspect and participate in a dialogue.

A diabetes educator who has a background in wellness would also find this manual a very important part of his or her toolkit.

Finally the manual could be partnered with your health-care provider as you use this tool as one of the ways of educating yourself about diabetes.

If you are like a growing number of individuals who are seeking more for their long-term health and want to take the next step, you can get more information about how you can do just this by contacting me on my website (www.askdoctoreno.com).

It is my hope that this manual will serve as a daily resource in answering some of the questions and that it will enrich your life's journey.

Eno A. Nsima-Obot, MD
Board Certified Internal Medicine & Well-Being Coach
WellCare Physician Services, Inc.

Acknowledgments

This manual has been a long time coming. I would like to acknowledge Ms. Shirley Hightower, a long-time patient and friend who encouraged me to start writing and believed that I had a message that was worth sharing.

My dear friend, Patrick Ebri, and my brother, Chris Akpan, for taking the time to review the manuscript to make certain that it was written in a way that conveyed easy understanding.

Miss Imogene Gonzalez, a graduate of Central Junior High School, class of 2010 Evergreen Park, Illinois, who so kindly provided the illustrations.

My thanks go to my virtual assistant, Ms. Amy Sanders, whose tireless edits and coordination saw this book to final completion and publishing.

My former life coach, Maren Perry, who held me accountable to "declare and fulfill" the completion of this book and always reflected my essence and limitless possibility.

Finally, the world's finest ICF-accredited coach-training program, Accomplishment Coaching, for providing me with the priceless gift of personal transformation that has lead to a new career path as a transformational speaker and life coach.

Thanks to you all.

What Is Diabetes?

You have just left your doctor's office, and you have just been informed that you have diabetes. You've heard of diabetes before, and you have a rough idea of what it means. You probably know a few people who have diabetes—some may even be relatives—but you never thought that it could happen to you!

Diabetes is a disorder in which the body is no longer able to handle blood sugar. Blood sugars are regulated by a hormone called insulin, which is released from an organ called the pancreas. When there is a defect in the way that insulin is released or any problem with the action of insulin with the cells of the body, the sugars remain in the bloodstream. This is called hyperglycemia (high blood sugar).

There are two main types of diabetes—type I and type II diabetes.

Type I diabetes is also called Insulin-dependent diabetes. It usually is genetic and is typically diagnosed at a very young age.

Type II diabetes is more common than type I diabetes, and it is commonly called non-insulin-dependent diabetes. It usually occurs at an older age. However, with the current obesity epidemic, and due to changes in our dietary habits, individuals are being diagnosed at a much younger age, sometimes even in the teenage years.

This manual is mainly for people with type II diabetes. No doubt

Eno Nsima-Obot, M.D.

those with type I can learn a lot about how to manage their diabetes, but my broad audience is type II diabetes patients.

The Relationship between Diabetes and Insulin

Insulin is a hormone produced in the pancreas by the beta cells. It is responsible for a variety of functions, most importantly coordinating the use of sugars and fats in order to produce an energy source for the body. Insulin secretion is dependent on a balance between blood sugar levels in the fasting state and after eating. When one is fasting, insulin stimulates the release of stored fat as a form of fuel for the body to function. After one eats (post-prandial state), insulin secretion is increased by the increased amount of glucose. This promotes the storage of excess sugars as triglycerides in the fat cells.

With time the body's cells become resistant to the effects of insulin. A condition called insulin resistance. The pancreas is doing what it normally does, releasing insulin, but the insulin is unable to be taken into the cells where it acts to break down sugars.

I like to compare this to "the landlord" changing the "door lock" (the cell receptors) on the tenant (the insulin). Insulin no longer works as well as it used to. The body's cells send a message back to the pancreas requesting that it release more insulin, and still, the locks stay "jammed" (insulin resistance).

In the end, we have a downward spiral of high blood sugar levels, high levels of insulin circulating in the bloodstream, and starving cells! Next, the liver gets a message that there is not enough sugar for the cells, and now the liver cells start to send out more sugar by the breaking down sugar stores called glycogen.

If this continues for a long time, the undetected blood sugars rise so high that a person may begin to develop symptoms.

Common symptoms of diabetes include the following:

- Extreme thirst
- Extreme hunger
- Frequent urination
- Blurred vision
- Extreme fatigue

2

- Weight loss

Other more subtle symptoms that may act as a warning of pre-diabetes include the following:

- Frequent yeast infections in women
- Frequent boils or abscesses
- Dark velvety areas over the creases of the skin called "acanthosis nigricans"

At times, the diagnosis of diabetes may be made quite early with the help of a blood test, and so the symptoms above may not have time to develop. Usually by the time that you begin to develop the symptoms listed above, you may have had diabetes for up to *five years!*

How Is Diabetes Diagnosed?

Diabetes is detected with a fasting blood sugar test. This could be done as part of an annual physical examination or a health screening. To obtain an accurate result, the blood test should be performed after an eight-to-twelve-hour fast. Normal fasting blood sugar levels should be less than 99 mg/dl. If the readings are above 100 mg/dl but less than 140 mg/dl, then this is called *impaired fasting glucose.*

When the fasting blood sugar levels are above 126 mg/dl, your doctor may recommend an *oral glucose tolerance test.* This test is performed over a two-hour period. You are required to fast for at least eight to twelve hours prior to the test. When you arrive at the lab, a fasting blood test is performed, and then you are given 75G of glucose (sucrose) to drink. After two hours, a repeat blood test is done. If the level is more than 200 mg/dl, then you are diagnosed with diabetes.

In my clinical practice, I used this test to diagnose borderline and frank diabetes even at mildly elevated fasting levels.

The current recommendations by the American Diabetes Association are that there be at least another repeat test, such as an elevated fasting sugar, on a separate day to confirm the diagnosis of diabetes. This may be a finger stick fasting glucose test done while you are at your doctor's office. It does not have to be a repeat of the oral glucose tolerance test.

What Is Borderline Diabetes?

Pre-diabetes or "borderline diabetes" is when the oral glucose tolerance test shows blood sugar levels less than 200 mg/dl but over 140 mg/dl. This indicates that there is a high likelihood that you could develop diabetes if you do not make some changes to your lifestyle.

Most recently, the American Diabetes Association approved the use of the A1C test to screen for diabetes. For more information about the A1C test, please refer to the chapter on "G-Glycosylated Hemoglobin."

Long-Term Complications of Type II Diabetes

There are two major types of complications associated with type II diabetes. They are divided into macrovascular complications and also microvascular complications.

It is beyond the scope of this manual to go into a description of the complications associated with diabetes; however, I believe it is also important to know what they are.

Macrovascular complications affect the major vessel beds of the body, including the following:

- The heart vessels, causing coronary artery disease
- The brain, causing cerebrovasular disease
- The peripheral circulation, causing peripheral vascular disease

The common reason for the development of these complications is *atherosclerosis,* which is the buildup of cholesterol plaques in the blood vessels.

Atherosclerosis begins earlier, and plaque builds up faster than it does in people without diabetes.

There are other associated diseases and conditions called "risk factors" that increase the risk for macrovascular complications:

- Hypertension

- Obesity (particularly central obesity, which is fat around the belly)
- Smoking
- Inadequate exercise

Microvascular complications associated with diabetes affect smaller vessels and include the following:

- Diabetic Retinopathy (eye disease)
- Diabetic Nephropathy (kidney disease)
- Diabetic Neuropathy (nerve diseases)

Diabetes and its associated complications are the fourth leading cause of death and disability in the United States.

The good news is that research shows that by controlling the blood sugars and keeping them within the recommended range, microvascular complications can be reduced.

So now that we know all this let's dive into the Diabetic Alphabet soup and learn how you too can live a more powerful life with Diabetes. Enjoy!

A—Acceptance

For a lot of people, being diagnosed with diabetes is a life-changing and mind-altering experience. It may also come with a sense of loss of what was felt like to be "healthy." All of a sudden, you are labeled with a medical disease, and now you have to start seeing a doctor on a regular basis to stay healthy. You may also experience a sense of loss because now you have to make certain dietary changes.

Either way, loss is hard to deal with and requires acceptance.

Without acceptance, all the other steps outlined in this manual are worthless. They just remain words on paper without relevance. It is only when action is attached to awareness and education that personal growth occurs.

With acceptance that you have diabetes, you can then arm yourself with the willpower to move forward (awareness). You can empower yourself with the knowledge that you need to make healthier decisions for yourself (action).

With acceptance comes self-love and also self-responsibility. Self-love means that you choose to embrace yourself as complete and resourceful and whole just as you are right now. It means that you have the right answers inside of you and all you need to do is commit to finding what works best for you. Self-responsibility (response-ability) means that you have the capacity to respond in a way that will make your life better. In other words, you make choices that cause better outcomes for you.

When self-love and self-responsibility are combined together, they create a powerful catalyst for change.

By accepting that you have diabetes, you are giving yourself a choice to make decisions early enough to alter any potential for a bad outcome.

Acceptance now becomes a chance at a new lease on life!

With acceptance, you are ready to stretch and grow in new directions that you had never thought possible. You become a *walking question mark* ready to search for the right answers and situations that work for you.

Journal Entry

Exercise 1 (a lesson in acceptance)

Look in a mirror for this exercise. Place your hands over your heart and say the following out loud: "I am the perfect expression of myself! There is no one else like me, and so I accept full responsibility for being me!"

Now write in your journal or the space below:

"Being diagnosed with diabetes means _____ to me."

B—Believe that You Can Live with Diabetes

Once you *accept* the diagnosis of diabetes, the next step is to begin to take action to begin living with diabetes.

The rest of this manual will only be useful to you if you have embraced acceptance and belief. Without acceptance and a strong unshakeable belief that *you can* make the changes in your lifestyle and move forward, then the rest of what I write about in this manual is only theoretical and words on a page with no relevance to your life.

In my years of practice, I have come across a number of patients who were under the misguided impression that if they accepted that they had diabetes, they were laying claim to a disease that would only have a negative impact on their lives. I have seen countless individuals take that attitude and return years later in a worse state than they were in when they were initially diagnosed.

This is simply because they were not willing to accept and then act!

I have also been fortunate to take care of patients who accepted their diagnosis and then partnered with me to find ways that could make them better.

By partnering with your health-care provider (and several other resources outlined under the chapter S—Support), you move yourself toward a higher level of well-being, which is the ultimate goal of this manual.

Journal Entry

Exercise 2 (declaration on belief)

Take a clean sheet of paper and write out the following declaration: "I live a full and healthy life with diabetes!"

Post this in several places that you can see and read this statement back to yourself several times a day.

This is a declaration, and it is a powerful tool that is designed to give your subconscious mind the permission to accept what it is that you are focusing on and now work to provide you with the tools to live a better life.

Denial is not healthy and uses up too much negative energy.

Believe that you can live a full and rewarding life despite the fact that you have been diagnosed with diabetes. Believe that the energies of the universe will align themselves with your soul. Then you open yourself to so much more potential and possibility in your life.

C—Commit to Change

Once you have accepted and believe that you can live a healthy life with diabetes, the next step is to commit to living that lifestyle.

As humans, our nature is to jump straight into action, oftentimes without adequate preparation. This is why we end up "falling off the wagon" despite our best efforts and never committing to lasting change.

There are several stages involved in making lasting lifestyle changes. It may be helpful to have a working knowledge of these stages so that you do not get discouraged if at first you do not succeed.

This is a brief outline of the different stages in the change process.

The Stages of Change

Pre-contemplation

The first stage of change is a stage called *pre-contemplation*. Simply put, change is not even on your radar screen. You may have thought about it very briefly—you may have decided not to eat too many sweets—but it's not something that you truly have any intention of going though with.

Contemplation

The next stage of the change process is called *contemplation*.

A typical example of this stage is when you have been to the doctor and you've been informed that your blood sugar levels are running outside of the target range. You are beginning to think that maybe you do need to make changes to your lifestyle, but you are nowhere near action; however, the thoughts of making healthier lifestyle choices are on your "radar screen," so to speak.

Preparation

After the contemplation stage is the stage of *preparation*. In this stage, you are getting ready for action by putting things in place. For instance, you may decide that you will no longer have cookies and ice cream for dessert but want to find other healthy replacements that will satisfy your sweet tooth. This is a good stage in the change process to make a list of things that you intend to do. An important thing that we fail to realize is that without a road map that clearly marks our destination, there is a chance that we just may not reach the destination.

It is worthwhile for you to spend a considerable amount of time in preparation so that you can come up with a concrete plan that is unique for you rather than adapt a cookie-cutter approach or follow what another person may have told you worked well for them.

Preparation lays the solid foundation for the next stage—action.

Action

Action is the stage that we are all very familiar with. Action makes us feel we are accomplishing a goal. However, when the proper steps have not been taken prior to action, then the action steps may not be as effective and may not produce lasting change. A common reason why people tend to fail- despite their heartfelt intentions to live a healthy lifestyle- is that they did not spend enough time in the contemplation and preparation phase but just jumped straight into action.

Relapse

Relapse is a stage to be aware of. Relapse is not unusual, and it happens. It can occur even to the well-prepared. A lot of people simply stop trying because they feel that they have failed when they go back to an old habit. That fear of failure stops them in their tracks, and they do not try again. Relapse can happen more than once.

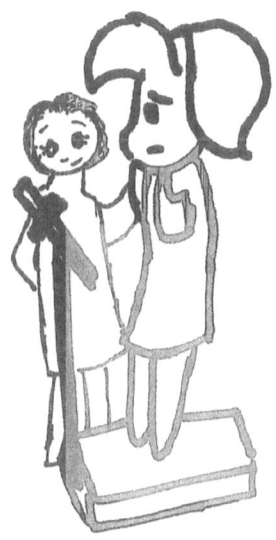

We see striking examples of this happening in a person who is attempting to quit smoking. Remember that it is okay to fall, get back up on your feet, and try again. But it is important to be aware of the *triggers* that caused the relapse.

One of the most challenging times during the year comes around the holiday season from Halloween all the way to New Year's Day. This is a time of the year when there is such an abundance of sweets, candies, and rich desserts adorning almost every dining table or gathering. Even for people who are not diabetic, the holidays are a time where a lot of people gain a few pounds in weight.

There are lessons to be learned even in the relapse phase. For instance, if you tend to relapse during the holidays and eat more desert and sweets at holiday parties, perhaps you could come up with measures to counter that urge. A good example would be making a commitment to increase the amount of exercise.

Maintenance

In the maintenance phase, we gain new skills to maintain the change in our lives. Most times, the new change has become a habit, and it is something that we are now able to do without too much effort or thought. During this phase, you are still working to prevent relapses, and so, you still need to be extra vigilant. Typically, the maintenance phase lasts anywhere from a few months up to five years.

Termination

This phase is synonymous to having *mastered* a habit or made a permanent change in your behavior. You have no temptation to resume an undesirable habit, or you are well on your way to living a healthier lifestyle.

The Benefits of Being Aware of the Stages of Change

I have taken the time to outline the stages of change as a way to provide more insight into why a lot of people tend to fail to make lasting changes despite their best intentions.

When you are aware of where you are in the change process, it allows you more insight into how to make lifelong changes rather than those that are transient or sporadic.

As stated earlier, the reason why a lot of people fail at making permanent healthy changes to their lifestyle despite their best intention is that they jump straight into the action phase without spending time in the preparation phase.

For instance, your doctor may recommend that you lose ten pounds in order to achieve better control of your blood sugars. You may jump straight into an exercise program and then find that you are not able to keep up with it a few weeks later.

Knowing about these stages allows you an honest self assessment, that allows you to prioritize which areas in your life you are willing to make changes to now, versus areas you are still contemplating making changes to. In other words, what matters most to you now?

It will also allow you to have the correct mindset when there are setbacks, as they are bound to occur. That is a part of life!

Simply being aware of what you are willing to do is also an equally powerful tool.

D—Drugs

If you are on medications, it is very important to know the names of the medications and specifically why you are taking them. There are several medications that are used in the treatment of diabetes. This is an overview of the common classes of drugs at the time of this writing and how they work.

Sulfonylureas

These are the oldest class of medications used to treat diabetes. They act on the beta cells of the pancreas to stimulate the release of more insulin. Because they are the oldest class of drugs, they are also the more affordable types of treatment. Recent guidelines issued by the American Diabetes Association no longer recommend that these drugs be considered as the first line of drugs to treat diabetes.

Examples of medications in this class include glyburide (Micronase and Diabeta) glipizide (Glucotrol) and glimepiride (Amaryl).

Secretagogues

These drugs also act on the beta cells to stimulate the release of insulin. The difference between secretagogues and the sulfonylureas is that these drugs target the rise in the sugars after you eat (postprandial sugars). Your doctor may decide to prescribe a secretagogue if your sugars tend to rise after you eat.

Examples of secretagogues are repaglinide (Prandin) and nateglinide (Starlix).

Thiazolidinediones

These drugs act at the level of the cells. They stimulate certain receptors on the cells called PPAR-y to increase the response of the cells to insulin. This leads to a reduction in the blood sugar levels.

Examples of this class of drugs are rosiglitazone (Avandia) and pioglitazone (Actos).

Biguanides

These drugs act by reducing the production of glucose by the liver. In diabetes, in spite of high circulating blood sugars, the liver continues to produce glucose from the breakdown of a substance called glycogen. Extensive studies document that biguanides help reduce the complications of diabetes that occur because of the damage to the large vessel complications (called macrovascular complications).

There is only one medication in this class, and it is called metformin (Glucophage).

Metformin also has a unique role in the prevention of progression to full blown diabetes, and it may be prescribed in pre-diabetes stages (commonly called borderline diabetes).

Alpha Glucosidase Inhibitors

Medications in this class prevent the absorption of carbohydrates from the intestines. This helps to preserve the beta cells in the pancreas.

Drugs in this class include acarbose (Precose) and miglitol (Glyset).

Dipeptidyl Peptidase (DPP)-4 Inhibitors

These are a new class of drugs. They act by deactivating enzymes called incretins which are found in the stomach and intestines. Incretins act in two ways: First, they increase the release of insulin from the pancreas. This action is similar to some of the other class of drugs that we have reviewed. In addition, they also shut down the release of glucagon. By doing this, the liver stops producing glucose from the glycogen stores.

DPP-4 inhibitors combine the function of secretagogues and also biguanides into one.

Examples of the DPP-4 inhibitors are sitagliptin (Januvia) and more recently saxagliptin (Onglyza).

Bile Acid Sequestrants

Bile acid sequestrants have been used to lower cholesterol for a long time. In recent clinical studies, they were also found to have an additional benefit of reducing A1C levels. It is not certain how they are able to do this, but they do have a benefit in helping in the reduction of the LDL cholesterol.

The drug in this class is called colesevelam (Welchol). Recently, Welchol was released as a powder that can be easily mixed in water, and it may be a lot easier than taking the six required pills per day!

GLP1 Mimetics

These drugs have several mechanisms of action. They copy the action of the incretin enzymes. They also suppress the release of glucagon—another way that it reduces the release of glucose. They also act by delaying the emptying of the stomach contents. In this way, you feel fuller for longer and so eat less.

The benefit of a class of drugs that has several mechanisms of action is that by acting on several pathways, it is likely to be more effective than drugs that only act on one pathway.

The drug in this class is called exenatide (Byetta). Recently, another drug, called Victoza, was added to this class .

These medications are administered by injection only. I found that to be a drawback for some individuals who may have hang-ups about injections or being labeled as someone on insulin.

Amylinomimetics

Amylin is an enzyme secreted along with insulin from the pancreatic cells. It has similar benefits to the GLP-1 mimetics. This drug is approved for people with type I diabetes as well as individuals with type II diabetes who require insulin but are still not well controlled on their current regimen. This drug also has an off-label benefit of promoting weight loss.

Pramlintide (Seemly) is available also as an injection.

Insulin

As type II diabetes progresses, at times insulin may be required. This is because as time goes on, the pancreas is no longer able to keep up with the increasing amounts of insulin required to maintain glucose control.

So in order to maintain glucose levels in the normal range and reduce the complications possible from poorly controlled diabetes, insulin may be required.

If your physician recommends insulin, it is because it is needed at this stage in your treatment.

If you feel resistant to this recommendation, I encourage you to go back to the ABC phase of this book and apply the same principles of accepting, believing, and committing:

- *Accept* the information that you require insulin.
- *Believe* that you can make the adjustment to starting an insulin regimen.
- *Commit* to learning how to administer insulin and also make the adjustments to your lifestyle that you need to make.

There are several types of insulin and they are formulated to act for different lengths of time:

- *Short-acting insulin:* The onset of action is thirty to sixty minutes, and it can last up to eight hours.
- *Rapid-acting insulin:* Usually, this type of insulin begins to act within ten to fifteen minutes and can last up to about five hours.

Examples in this class would include insulin lispro (Humalog), insulin aspart (Novolog), and insulin glulisine (Apidra).

Other types of insulin are:

- *Intermediate-acting insulin:* Onset of action occurs within one to three hours, and its effect lasts a lot longer than the rapid-acting insulin, namely up to eighteen hours. NPH is the only intermediate acting insulin.
- *Long-acting insulin analogues:* This class of insulin analogues starts to act within one to three hours, and their effects last up to twenty-four hours.

Examples from this class include insulin glargine (Lantus) and also insulin determir (Levemir).

There is also premixed insulin. These types of insulin come in a premixed combination. They are very beneficial for the person who has an active lifestyle or perhaps for an older person who may have difficulty taking multiple injections a day.

They are a combination of intermediate, long-acting insulin, and rapid-acting insulin.

Premixed insulin combinations attempt to mimic the way that the pancreas releases insulin. After a meal, there is an immediate surge in insulin release to take care of the postprandial sugar rise and then a low basal level of insulin that occurs throughout the day.

Examples of combinations are as follows:

70/30 (70% NPH and 30% regular)

50/50 (50% NPH and 50% regular)

*Novolog Mix 70/30

*Humalog Mix 75/25

*Humalog Mix 50/50

Insulin is available in vials as well as a prefilled pen. This makes it easier to carry around and administer discretely.

Insulin should be refrigerated in order to maintain its potency. Once taken out of the refrigerator, it can be left at room temperature for thirty days. It is important to avoid extremely high and low temperatures. Insulin should never be placed in a freezer.

Insulin is easy to self-administer, and you can learn how to do this in a short time. It is injected with a very small needle just under the skin.

What Are the Best Sites to Inject Insulin?

The best site to inject the insulin is the anterior abdomen, namely the belly. This is because there is more subcutaneous tissue and the insulin gets absorbed faster from this site. Because it has such a large surface area, it is easier to rotate the areas where you inject.

The thighs, deltoid (upper arm), and the buttocks are less reliable sites, because the insulin gets absorbed a little more slowly from these sites. Avoid injecting into your thigh or arm if you plan to exercise soon after, as this will affect the rate at which the insulin is absorbed and may cause erratic drops in your blood sugars.

The medications listed above are not an exhaustive list of all the medications used to treat diabetes. You may have other medical conditions, such as hypertension or heart disease, and your doctor may have put you on more medications.

It is very important to keep a medication list of all the drugs that you are taking. Be sure to include the medications that specialists may have prescribed for you as well.

Some Important Tips

Be aware of potential side effects.

Be certain to get a list of the potential side effects from the pharmacist. If you experience any of the listed side effects, stop the medication immediately and call your physician.

Check to see whether to take your medications with food.

You may need to take most of the medications with food. This is particularly important with insulin and also the oral medications. If you fail to do this, you may be at risk for a sudden drop in blood sugars called hypoglycemia, which can be potentially life threatening.

Check with the pharmacist about potential drug interactions.

Be sure to verify from the pharmacist whether there is any potential for multiple drug interactions. These interactions can range from minimal to life-threatening effects. If there is a potential problem, be sure to alert your doctor immediately.

Have your medications filled at the same pharmacy.

It is best to have *all* your medications filled at the same pharmacy. This is important so that your pharmacist can alert your doctor about potential drug reactions as stated above. "Bargain shopping" for your medications at different locations may have life-threatening effects. If you *have* to shop for bargain prices, be sure to give every pharmacist a list of *all* the medications that you are taking. Be sure to include supplements that you may also be taking. (Refer to the chapter on supplements for more information on this topic.)

Action Steps

Make a list of your current medications. If you are not certain why you are taking a certain medication, contact your doctor's office and find out why, or you could even inquire from the pharmacist.

Write a note about why you are taking the medications next to the name of each. It would be a good idea to laminate this list at a local print center like Kinko's so that it does not fade.

The medication list serves several purposes: First of all, it lets your doctors know what medications and current dosages you are currently on.

It is also important to let your family members know the medications that you are on. Be certain to let your family members know where you keep a list of your medications so that they can access this in the event of an emergency.

Here is an example of what the list should look like:

Glyburide 5 mg two times a day
Reason: to help control blood sugar

Lipitor 20 mg once a day at bedtime
Reason: to help control cholesterol

Humalog 75/25 twice daily with breakfast and dinner
Reason: to also help control blood sugar

E—Exercise

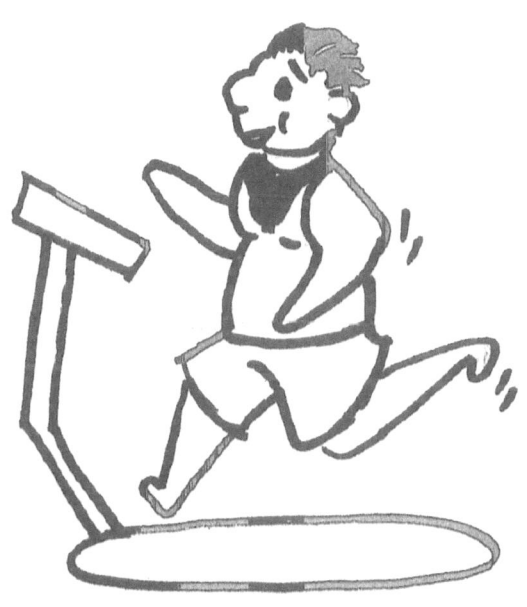

Before you start any exercise program, consult your physician for a full physical examination. It is also recommended that you undergo cardiac stress testing if you are diabetic and over the age of forty.

According to the surgeon general and other authorities on exercise and physical activity, current recommendations are to incorporate thirty minutes of physical activity at least five days a week.

Exercise is an important component of living a healthy lifestyle. As adults we tend to approach exercise with trepidation and not look at it as a fun activity.

With diabetes, exercise has been documented to help better control blood sugars.

Starting an Exercise Program

When the majority of people think of exercise, they associate this with only aerobic exercise. However, a well-balanced exercise regimen includes five components.

- *Aerobic exercise* (also known as cardiovascular exercise)
- *Resistance exercise* (also known as weight training)
- *Stretching exercise* (also known as static exercise)
- *Balance Training*
- *Core Stability*

Do not focus on only one component to the exclusion of the others.

A reasonable ratio would be 60 percent aerobic exercise, 40 percent resistance training, stretching, balance, and core stability. Depending on your level of physical fitness and overall fitness goals, you may vary that ratio.

For instance, if you are under emotional stress or your muscles are sore or tight from a previous workout, you may want to incorporate more stretching exercises for the next few days.

Aerobic exercise is any physical activity that raises the heart rate by increasing the pumping action of the heart muscle.

It is important to exercise within the accepted heart rate for your age.

For aerobic activity, the recommended heart rate is between 60 to 80 percent of the *maximum heart rate* for your age.

The maximum heart rate is calculated by subtracting your age from 220.

For instance, if you are fifty years old, your maximum heart rate is 170. When you exercise between 60 to 80 percent of your maximum heart rate, your heart rate on your heart rate monitor should read between 102 and 144 beats per minute.

Do not attempt to exercise any higher than 60 to 80 percent of your maximum heart rate. If you notice that your heart rate is higher, cut back on the intensity of your exercise.

Below are examples of moderate physical activity. It includes the length of time that it would take to burn a thousand calories per week. In order to lose one pound a week, you will need to burn 2,100 calories per week.

Examples of Moderate Physical Activity

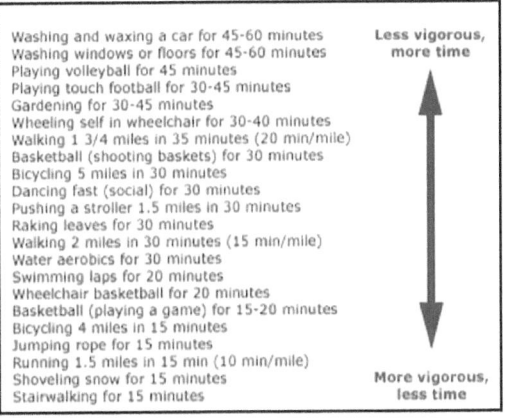

Washing and waxing a car for 45-60 minutes — Less vigorous, more time
Washing windows or floors for 45-60 minutes
Playing volleyball for 45 minutes
Playing touch football for 30-45 minutes
Gardening for 30-45 minutes
Wheeling self in wheelchair for 30-40 minutes
Walking 1 3/4 miles in 35 minutes (20 min/mile)
Basketball (shooting baskets) for 30 minutes
Bicycling 5 miles in 30 minutes
Dancing fast (social) for 30 minutes
Pushing a stroller 1.5 miles in 30 minutes
Raking leaves for 30 minutes
Walking 2 miles in 30 minutes (15 min/mile)
Water aerobics for 30 minutes
Swimming laps for 20 minutes
Wheelchair basketball for 20 minutes
Basketball (playing a game) for 15-20 minutes
Bicycling 4 miles in 15 minutes
Jumping rope for 15 minutes
Running 1.5 miles in 15 min (10 min/mile)
Shoveling snow for 15 minutes — More vigorous, less time
Stairwalking for 15 minutes

A moderate amount of physical activity is roughly equivalent to physical activity that uses approximately 150 calories (kcal) of energy per day or a thousand calories per week. Some activities can be performed at various intensities. The suggested durations correspond to the expected intensity of effort.

(Source: Up to date Patient Information on exercise www.uptodate. com)

This list just serves as a guide, so get creative and think of more activities that you would like to do. Include daily activities, such as gardening, washing the windows, or scrubbing the floors. Also, walking the dog can be a great form of activity. Remember, you will want a regimen that you are most likely to stick to, so add lots of variety.

Resistance Training

Resistance training is exercise that leads to increasing muscle size and mass. When you increase muscle mass, you burn calories faster *even in between workouts!* Resistance training has the additional benefit of reducing bone loss, which can lead to a condition called osteoporosis in postmenopausal women.

Most exercise guidelines recommend incorporating resistance training *at least two to three times a week*. It is also important not to work out the same muscle groups two days in a row. For instance, work out the upper body on one day—this may include the arms, chest, and upper back—and then work the lower body the next time (lower back, thighs, and legs). Abdominal exercises are one group of resistance exercises that can be done daily, depending on their intensity. If you have a doubt about incorporating daily abdominal exercises, then consult a personal trainer.

If you have a gym membership, weight machines are a great tool. You can also do resistance training at home with bar bells, kettle bells, and resistance bands, or you can help while you use your own body weight in the form of abdominal crunches, lunges, squats, and push-ups. Get really creative if you are working out at home. You can use soup cans or kegs of water.

Stretching

Most aerobic and strength training exercises cause the muscles to contract and stiffen. This can affect overall flexibility. Stretching improves the range of motion of your joints and the posture. It is very important to include stretching exercises before and after workouts. Most personal trainers and exercise physiologists may recommend a brief warm-up before you stretch in order to avoid damaging the muscles and the ligaments.

Core Stability Exercises

The core muscles are the muscles located in your abdomen, back, and pelvis, and they are responsible for your posture. Maintaining a strong core becomes very important as we begin to age, because it helps to keep the posture upright, preventing the development of kyphosis, which is a curving of the spine. Core exercises also help maintain balance and reduce the potential for falls, especially in the elderly.

Examples of core training would include exercises like back- and abdominal-strengthening exercises.

Balance Training

As we age, we may begin to lose our balance. This puts us at risk of falls which could result in bone fractures.

Traditionally, diabetes tends to affect older people, and it is important to maintain good balance by incorporating balance training as part of your exercise regimen.

A bonsu ball, yoga poses, Pilates, and Tai Chi can help with balance training and also core training.

A Special Note about Yoga, Pilates, and Tai Chi

If I were to recommend any particular form of exercise that incorporated *all* components of a well-balanced exercise program, it would be yoga, pilates, or tai chi.

In my experience, I have found that yoga can cover all aspects of an exercise program from cardiovascular and resistance training by the practice of a sequence of "asanas" to core and stability and balance in the "poses." Yoga, pilates, and tai chi all involve aligning the body, mind and spirit.

I would recommend that you start out in group classes in order to reduce the risk of injury and learn the correct form and breathing patterns that are associated with these practices. As you get more familiar with the different poses, you can start a home regimen.

Tips on Starting an Exercise Program

Start small.

Perhaps you have never exercised. It would be unrealistic to expect that you start at thirty minutes per day for five days per week! Once you identify an activity that you enjoy doing, your initial goal is to *start small.*

Go back to the chapter on commitment and review the stages of change. This is very important when you are taking on a new habit or changing an existing behavior.

For instance, if you decide that you would like to start a walking program and want to use a treadmill, start slow for a few days—maybe at a pace of two miles per hour or even slower. The goal is not to break a sweat at this pace but simply show up to the activity. This is a way of training your brain in a nonthreatening way to get used to this new activity.

Next, gradually begin to increase the speed and the amount of time that you walk. For instance, walk at a speed of four miles per hour for five to ten minutes.

Each week, you can gradually increase your pace and also the length of time until you reach your goal of at least thirty minutes a day.

Chart your progress each week. This is a great motivational tool, and it also provides important feedback.

Make exercise a habit.

It's been a longstanding debate about exactly how long it takes to truly develop a habit, but *consistent action* for *at least twenty-one days* is a good starting point. Don't worry. Just commit to consistent action, and the results will follow.

In a month or two, you will be well on your way to incorporating more physical activity into your life.

Consistent exercise has been found to help maintain healthy blood sugars. In fact there are some people with diabetes who are able to control their blood sugars with exercise and diet alone. They are a small segment of diabetics but it still is possible. In other words, they do not need to take any medications.

Diabetes is caused by many factors that can be modified by a change in lifestyle. Regrettably, many people are not willing to do what it takes to make lifestyle adjustments, citing reasons like "lack of time," "a heavy work schedule," "just not motivated," "it's too hard," and myriad other reasons.

Your physician can determine if this is a reasonable option for you. It is important to make sure that you pay meticulous attention to your blood sugars if you are using diet and exercise alone to control your blood sugars.

Important Tools for an Exercise Program

Heart-Rate Monitor

I recommend a good quality heart-rate monitor whenever you are exercising. This is important to determine your heart rate and also to ensure than you are exercising within 60 to 80 percent of your maximal heart rate.

Comfortable Athletic Shoes

Comfortable athletic shoes are a very important part of a physical exercise regimen. It is a worthwhile investment to go to a reputable sports store to purchase a quality pair. If possible, get a gait analysis performed. Be certain to change your sneakers every five hundred miles. This includes mileage if you use your shoes to do other things in addition to exercise. To cut back on this, I usually recommend having a pair of shoes dedicated to exercise and then a pair that is used to run errands.

Pedometer

A pedometer is a counting device clipped to the waistline that counts the number of steps taken. A pedometer is a great tool to use every day as you go about your regular activity. It can be purchased from a sports shop, and it is very affordable. Get a basic model that simply counts steps, distance, and perhaps calories. Don't worry about "bells and whistles" on the device. The more functions it has, the more expensive it is likely to be (and the more likely that it may be a challenge to program). Be sure to follow the instructions and calibrate your pedometer to your gait before you start using it.

The Ten-Thousand-Steps-a-Day Program

This is a fun and creative way to get moving. There are a number of walking clubs that are pioneered after this program, including the ten-thousand-steps program as part of the fifty-million-pound challenge made popular by Dr. Ian Smith. On average, ten thousand steps per day is roughly equivalent to five miles per day.

Here's how to create your own thirty-day program: On day one, remember to *start small*. At the end of the day, review how many steps you have walked.

Let's say you walked three thousand steps in day one. The goal should be to increase by *at least* 250–500 steps each day. Gradually, continue to make a conscious effort to increase the number of steps that you walk each day. Remember, you are taking small steps each day.

Get comfortable shoes on, get a pedometer, and enter into your personal "ten-thousand-steps-a-day challenge!"

Action Steps

Make a list of three activities that you enjoy

1.

2.

3.

If you'd like, start a ten-thousand-steps-a-day club by inviting friends, colleagues at work, and family members to support you in getting physically active.

F—Foot Care

Regular foot care is an important part of your diabetes care.

As diabetes progresses, some individuals may develop diminished sensation in their feet. Your doctor should perform a simple test called a "fine filament test" at every visit. Just as the name suggests, it is a simple, *painless* test with a fine filament touching the tips of the toes. This test determines the health of the nerves in the feet. Diabetic neuropathy is one of the microvascular complications of diabetes.

Maintaining the health of the feet is important to your overall health as a diabetic. Check your feet every day, especially in between your toes. Take special care to dry in between your toes, and if they are moist, apply a foot powder to prevent *athlete's foot,* which is a fungal infection that occurs when moisture stays trapped in between the feet. A foot infection could cause the blood sugars to rise. Pay particular attention to any change in color, such as increased redness or darkened color, or even pain in your legs and feet. Bring this to the *immediate* attention of your primary care doctor.

Exercise caution when you cut the toenails. Do not cut the toenails too close to the skin, because this may cause damage to the nail bed and subsequent foot infections. If you get pedicures at a nail shop, be careful not to get your feet scraped with sharp objects. This can lead to small abrasions that could act as another entry point for foot infections.

When you are buying shoes, be sure that your toes are not tightly *cramped* in them. A good idea would be to buy wide fitting shoes if you encounter that problem.

Healthy feet allow you to move better. Be sure to have an annual foot check performed by a podiatrist to determine whether you require special fitting shoes or customized orthotics to fit into your shoes.

G—Glycosylated Hemoglobin

Glycosylated hemoglobin, also known as the A1C, is a blood screening test used to determine how well controlled the blood sugars have been over the prior six to eight weeks.

The glycosylated hemoglobin is determined by the fasting sugar levels and also sugar levels after you eat (postprandial glucose levels).

The goal is to keep the glycosylated hemoglobin *below* 7 percent. This is equivalent to blood sugar levels that are consistently less than 140 mg/dl.

The recommended target A1C by the American College of Endocrinologists is less than 6 percent, which correlates with sugars on average less than 100 mg/dl.

Know your A1C and work with your primary care doctor or endocrinologist to keep it less than 7 percent.

For every percentage point that your A1C rises above 7 percent, there is an exponential risk in the complications related to diabetes.

Perhaps you may have heard your doctor caution you about these potential complications. A lot of patients are under the misguided impression that once you are diagnosed with diabetes, it goes without saying that you will develop complications, no matter what you do.

By being proactive and partnering with your physician, the A1C can be maintained at less than 7 percent.

In my years of clinical practice, I had a large number of patients who were able to maintain their A1C at less than 7 percent and a smaller percentage who maintained an A1C less than 6 percent.

They are my walking ambassadors who are living proof that this can be done.

Because the two contributing factors to the A1C are both the fasting blood sugar levels and the blood sugar levels after you eat (postprandial sugar levels), I usually recommend that my patients check their sugars not only while they are fasting but also two hours after they eat a meal.

I use the recommendations by the American College of Endocrinology: The recommended range for fasting blood sugar levels is 80–120 mg/dl. The recommended levels two hours after you eat should be less than 140 mg/dl. (Please refer to the appendix for a sample of the instruction sheet I give to my patients.)

HbA1c	4.0	4.1	4.2	4.3	4.4	4.5	4.6	4.7	4.8	4.9
Glucose	65	69	72	76	79	83	86	90	93	97
HbA1c	5.0	5.1	5.2	5.3	5.4	5.5	5.6	5.7	5.8	5.9
Glucose	101	104	108	111	115	118	122	126	129	133
HbA1c	6.0	6.1	6.2	6.3	6.4	6.5	6.6	6.7	6.8	6.9
Glucose	136	140	143	147	151	154	158	161	165	168
HbA1c	7.0	7.1	7.2	7.3	7.4	7.5	7.6	7.7	7.8	7.9
Glucose	172	175	179	183	186	190	193	197	200	204
HbA1c	8.0	8.1	8.2	8.3	8.4	8.5	8.6	8.7	8.8	8.9
Glucose	207	211	215	218	222	225	229	232	236	240
HbA1c	9.0	9.1	9.2	9.3	9.4	9.5	9.6	9.7	9.8	9.9
Glucose	243	247	250	254	257	261	264	268	272	275
HbA1c	10.0	10.1	10.2	10.3	10.4	10.5	10.6	10.7	10.8	10.9
Glucose	279	282	286	289	293	297	300	304	307	311
HbA1c	11.0	11.1	11.2	11.3	11.4	11.5	11.6	11.7	11.8	11.9
Glucose	314	318	321	325	329	332	336	339	343	346
HbA1c	12.0	12.1	12.2	12.3	12.4	12.5	12.6	12.7	12.8	12.9

*Here is an A1C chart that gives a good illustration of the relationship between the A1C levels and blood glucose levels.

Source: Rohlfing, Curt L. BES; Hsiao-Mei Wiedmeyer, MS; Randie R. Little, PHD; Jack D. England; Alethea Tennill, MS; and David E. Goldstein, MD. "Defining the Relationship Between Plasma Glucose and HbA1c, Analysis of glucose profiles and HbA1c in the Diabetes Control and Complications Trial." Diabetes Care 25:275-278, 2002.

Action Steps

On your next visit to your primary care doctor, request to know what your glycosylated hemoglobin (A1C) is.

For a more visual analysis, I would recommend that you use the graph attached to chart your A1C. Keep in mind that your goal is to ensure that the A1C is below 7 percent, preferably less than 6 percent.

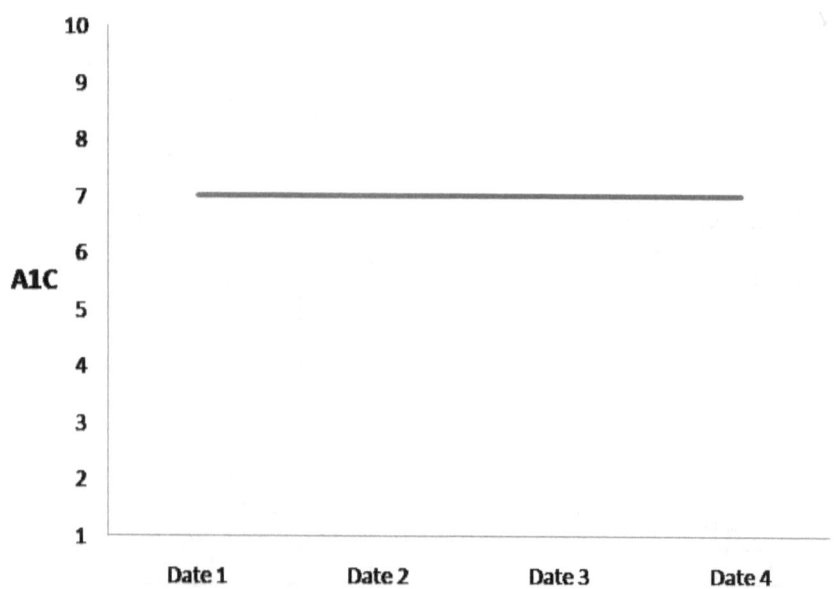

H—Heart Health and Hypertension

Individuals with type II diabetes mellitus are at twice the risk for developing heart disease compared to the general population. In addition, those who have a heart attack are more likely to have complications, such as heart failure or continued angina. Angina is chest pain caused by blockage of the arteries supplying blood to the heart.

The reason for the increased risk for heart disease is due to multiple factors that act at the level of the cells and lead to an increased tendency for the development of plaques and also clots in the blood vessels.

Some factors that can affect the progression of heart disease

Hypertension

Hypertension is also known as high blood pressure. Hypertension and diabetes can occur together. Blood pressure has two components to it—systolic and diastolic blood pressure. Systolic blood pressure refers to the pressure that is produced when the heart contracts and pushes blood out of the heart and into the blood vessels. The diastolic blood pressure is the pressure in the blood vessels when the heart relaxes. Think of the circulatory system as a municipal water system. The heart is the water pump sending water out into the pipes (the circulatory system) each time it pumps (the systolic pressure) and then receiving water back from the pipes (the blood vessels) to be pumped out again (the diastolic pressure).

When the pressure remains too high, this causes damage to the circulation and also the vital organs of the body, namely the kidneys (kidney failure), the brain (stroke), and the heart wall (heart failure). Research has shown that when sustained over a long period of time that blood pressures over 140/90 mm hg can cause damage.

In diabetes the goal is to reduce the blood pressure to 130/80 mm hg or less. For every 10 mm hg decrease in the systolic blood pressure (upper number), there is a 12 percent decreased risk of developing heart disease.

Hyperlipidemia

I have dedicated a chapter to lipids. High cholesterol levels increase the risk for cholesterol plaques, which can lead to heart disease. Some clinical studies have shown the long-term benefits of certain drugs called 'statin agents' in reducing heart disease.

Smoking

Smoking increases the risk of heart disease by raising the level of LDL cholesterol. When you stop smoking, this increased risk gradually goes down.

Elevated Blood Sugars

Sustained high blood sugars result in elevated A1C levels. With every 1 percent increase in A1C, there was a concurrent rise in the risk for heart disease. This is yet another reason why it is very important to control blood sugars well.

Sex (Gender)

Women who have diabetes have an increased risk of heart disease. This may be due to the fact that diabetes negates the beneficial effect a woman's hormones play in protecting her from heart disease before she goes through menopause. We're not entirely sure. But it's important that women are meticulous in ensuring that their blood sugars are well controlled.

Exercise

As I have outlined in another part of this manual, exercise has a multitude of benefits, including reducing the risk for heart disease in people diagnosed with diabetes.

Alcohol Intake

Contrary to what may be thought, moderate alcohol intake has been associated with a *reduced risk* for death from heart disease. The key here is *moderation.*

Action Steps

Some of the factors that I outlined in this chapter are "modifiable risk factors." In other words, you can make a change in these habits if you choose to. Examples would include smoking, exercise, and alcohol consumption.

Using the space here, make a list of some of the habits that you can commit to changing.

1. _____
2. _____
3. _____
4. _____
5. _____
6. _____
7. _____
8. _____
9. _____
10. _____

Now go back and review the chapter on commitment.

Next pick three habits that you will commit to changing in the next sixty-three days.

1. _____
2. _____
3. _____

Become aware of what stage of change you are in each of the three habits. For instance, if you smoke and you have never thought about quitting, then you are perhaps in the "precontemplation" phase. If you have just thought about starting an exercise program, then you are in the "contemplation phase."

Write out that steps that you will need to take to change these habits.

I—Immunizations

Immunizations are very important for people living with diabetes. They need to be reviewed as part of their annual preventive physical examination.

Below is a list of the current immunizations recommended by the Centers for Disease Control and Prevention:

Pneumococcal Vaccine

Pneumococcal disease is a very serious illness caused by bacteria called "streptococcus pneumoniae." This can result in serious infections like pneumonia in addition to a blood-borne illness called septicemia. In America, pneumococcal disease accounts for thousands of deaths each year.

Most of these fatal cases occur in people over the age of sixty-five years. The vaccine is usually recommended to those over sixty five years of age.

Tetanus-Diphtheria Toxoid

Tetanus is commonly called "lockjaw." It is caused by a bacterial poison (called a toxin) that affects the nervous system. Tetanus can be contracted through a cut or wound when it becomes contaminated with tetanus bacteria. The bacteria can get in through a tiny pinprick or even a scratch. Deep puncture wounds or cuts like those made by nails or knives also increase the risk for infection with tetanus. Tetanus bacteria are commonly found in soil, dust, and manure. Infection with tetanus causes severe muscle spasms and the "locking" of the jaw, which renders the person unable to open their mouth or swallow. Eventually, this leads to death by suffocation. Tetanus is not spread from person to person.

Diphtheria is a respiratory infection. Symptoms may include a sore throat, low-grade fever, and swollen neck glands. An individual may develop hoarseness and a runny nose.

Approximately 20 to 60 percent of adults develop an increased risk of developing diphtheria because of the waning of the protection that was provided by the vaccine earlier on in life.

Because of this, tetanus is usually given as a combined vaccine called tetanus-diphtheria and booster every ten years.

Influenza Vaccine

Influenza accounts for more than twenty thousand deaths in the United States each year. Death from influenza is usually at both extremes of life—the very young and the elderly.

H1N1 Vaccine

This vaccine is a recent one that has been added to the list of current vaccines. Persons with chronic medical conditions like diabetes should get the H1N1 vaccine. As there may be some concern about the fact that this is a relatively new vaccine and little may be known about the long-term effects, I encourage you to consult your physician to learn more about the vaccine and their recommendations.

Action Steps

Keep a record of your immunization shots just in case you are asked about it at another facility. For instance, if you get admitted to a hospital, most of the guidelines before discharge may include a pneumonia shot. If you keep a record of your shots, then you will be able to let your doctor know when you received the immunization.

J—Journal

A journal can be very revealing, as well as healing as you make discoveries in your journey toward living a powerful life with diabetes. Not everybody may feel comfortable with words, but the goal is not to make you a renowned author by any stretch of imagination.

Simply taking steps to make notes about how you are feeling on any particular day and then checking your glucose log to determine whether or not there are possible connections can be a great learning tool.

For instance, you may notice that your sugars run high when you are in a bad mood or stressed out. If you went a step further and kept a record of how you react when you are stressed, you may discover that you have an increased craving for sweets and instinctively reach into the candy jar sitting on a colleague's desk or that you have a double portion of dessert just to calm some of the anxiety that you may be feeling.

Keeping a journal this way may help you brainstorm more constructive ways of dealing with the stress, as well as being a conduit for stress release.

It also allows you to practice being responsible for how life goes for you. Ultimately journaling can create an opportunity to truly live more powerfully with diabetes.

Here are some other reasons for journaling such as:

- *A food journal* is a very effective tool, especially when you are newly diagnosed with diabetes or when you are embarking on a weight loss program.

- *A gratitude journal* can be very beneficial as you gain back your power and discover healthy ways to live with diabetes. Many people are initially upset and discouraged when they are diagnosed with diabetes. They may shut down and isolate themselves or even choose not to deal with their illness in an effective or constructive way.

By writing down things that we are grateful for each and every day, over time this helps to change the way that we view issues in our lives. Research has shown that the simple act of keeping a gratitude journal enhances overall well-being, and that people who keep them are better able to handle stress.

Action Steps

Buy a three subject notebook. Label one section "daily journal," the next section "food journal," and the third section "gratitude journal."

Do not feel pressured to write in every section every day. (But if you can, that would be awesome!)

Make it a habit to write under the daily journal or the food journal several times a week, or write in it if there is something striking that you may want to share with your doctor at your next visit. Keep your entries brief.

In the "gratitude section," spend at least five minutes on a select day in the evening before you go to bed. List at least five things that you are grateful for. Be creative and try not to repeat the same things every day. As you get used to journaling more, you may start to want to write in the gratitude journal every day.

At the end of twenty-one days, check in with yourself and see how writing in the gratitude journal has changed the way you feel.

Happy journaling!

K—Kindred History

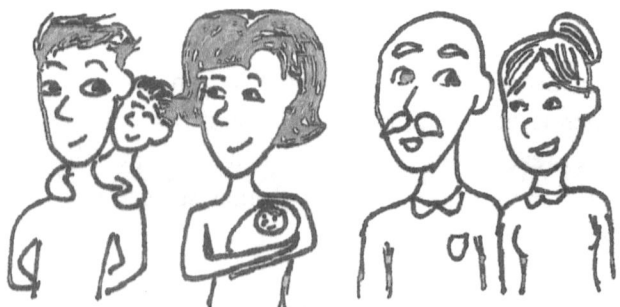

"Kindred" is another word for family. It is very important to know your family history, particularly as it relates to medical issues.

Certain medical conditions run in families. They may be hereditary, which means that you may have a greater propensity to these diseases even if there is not a genetic link. Or they may be genetic, which means that these diseases get transmitted through the genes.

When you are recording your family history, do this for both sides of your family—both your mother and father's side. It would also be optimal to collect medical histories from three generations, namely the first generation (children, siblings, and parents), second-degree relatives (aunts and uncles), and the third generation (grandparents).

There are certain diseases that tend to run in families, such as heart disease, susceptibility to strokes, certain cancers like breast, ovarian, prostate, and colon cancer, mental illnesses, osteoporosis, arthritis, obesity, and diabetes.

Here's an important fact about the importance of knowing your family history, particularly as it relates to diabetes: ***If one parent has type II diabetes, there's a 40 percent chance a child will develop type II diabetes. When both parents have it, the chances increase to 80 percent.***

If you know your family history, this hopefully increases your personal awareness so that you can begin to take preventive measures in your lifestyle.

It also helps to alert other family members, especially your children, so that they too can start making changes to their lifestyle. Make a commitment to improve the overall health of your family by doing things such as increasing physical activity, changing your diet and maintaining a healthy body weight.

Be proactive in your overall health. Start to collect a detailed family medical history today. Be open with your family members about any illnesses that you have. Encourage your family members to be open with you.

Too many times, family members appear oblivious to each other's medical illnesses or may learn too late to make changes in their lifestyle.

Think of the family medical history as a road map that the family collectively should take time to study and update in order to make a difference for future generations.

Action Steps

Use this page to write down the medical history of family members. You may notice that this is the same medical history that your doctor asks you about from time to time, especially during your annual health checkups.

Mother:

Alive/deceased
Diabetes Y/N
Hypertension Y/N
Stroke Y/N
Cancer Y/N (Please specify.)

_____

Mental illness Y/N (Please specify.)

_____

Arthritis Y/N (Please specify.)

_____

List any other medical illnesses

_____

Father:

Alive/deceased
Diabetes Y/N
Hypertension Y/N
Stroke Y/N
Cancer Y/N (Please specify.)

_____

Mental illness Y/N (Please specify.)

_____

Arthritis Y/N (Please specify.)

_____

List any other medical illnesses

_____

Mother's mother age ___
Alive/deceased
Diabetes Y/N
Hypertension Y/N
Stroke Y/N
Cancer Y/N (Please specify.)

_____

Mental illness Y/N (Please specify.)

_____

Arthritis Y/N (Please specify.)

_____

List any other medical illnesses

_____

Mother's father age___
Alive/deceased
Diabetes Y/N
Hypertension Y/N
Stroke Y/N
Cancer Y/N (Please specify.)

_____

Mental illness Y/N (Please specify.)

_____

Arthritis Y/N (Please specify.)

_____

List any other medical illnesses

_____

Father's mother age____
Alive/deceased
Diabetes Y/N
Hypertension Y/N
Stroke Y/N
Cancer Y/N (Please specify.)

_____

Mental illness Y/N (Please specify.)

_____

Arthritis Y/N (Please specify.)

_____

List any other medical Illnesses

_____

Father's father age____
Alive/deceased
Diabetes Y/N
Hypertension Y/N
Stroke Y/N
Cancer Y/N (Please specify.)

_____

Mental illness Y/N (Please specify.)

_____

Arthritis Y/N (Please specify.)

_____

List any other medical illnesses

_____

_____

Any other significant medical history in mother's relatives:
Diabetes Y/N
Hypertension Y/N
Stroke Y/N
Cancer Y/N (Please specify.)

_____

Mental illness Y/N (Please specify.)

_____

Arthritis Y/N (Please specify.)

_____

Any other significant medical history in father's relatives:
Diabetes Y/N
Hypertension Y/N
Stroke Y/N
Cancer Y/N (Please specify.)

_____

Mental illness Y/N (Please specify.)

_____

Arthritis Y/N (Please specify.)

_____

Children:
Diabetes Y/N
Hypertension Y/N
Stroke Y/N
Cancer Y/N (Please specify.)

_____

Mental illness Y/N (Please specify.)

_____

Arthritis Y/N (Please specify.)

_____

Other notes:

_____

L—Lipid Levels

Lipids are the fats in the body. They serve many functions in the body, the most important being that they are a source of energy for the cells. They also form part of the wall of living cells called membranes. Lipids are also important in the transport of certain substances like vitamins. They also play an important function in the formation of body chemicals called hormones. There is no doubt that lipids play a role in maintaining overall health.

Hyperlipidemia

Hyperlipidemia is the medical term used to describe excess lipids in the body.

There are several classes of lipids. The most common classes are the total cholesterol, LDL cholesterol, HDL cholesterol, and triglycerides.

It is important to know the different classes of the lipid profile. I use the following terms to describe them for my patients:

- *LDL—Lousy cholesterol*
- *HDL—Happy cholesterol*
- *Triglycerides*—The fatty substance present in the bloodstream

In the chapter on heart health and hypertension, I stated that being diagnosed with diabetes puts you at *twice* the risk of developing heart disease. High cholesterol levels increase the risk of developing heart disease, because they contribute to the development of plaque, which causes a narrowing of the arteries.

A *fasting lipid panel* is a simple blood test ordered by your doctor. In order for it to be accurate, it needs to be done after at least an eight-to-ten-hour fast.

Here are the recommended cholesterol goals to be aware of as a diabetic by the National Cholesterol Education Panel:

> **LDL cholesterol less than 70 optimal**
>
> **Less than 100 mg/dl acceptable**
>
> **HDL cholesterol more than 40 mg/dl acceptable**
>
> **More than 60 mg/dl optimal**
>
> **Triglycerides less than 150 mg/dl acceptable**
>
> **Total Cholesterol less than 190 mg/dl**

Several lifestyle measures can be taken to maintain healthy lipid levels. These include an optimal diet and exercise program.

I believe that commitment to embracing these lifestyle changes are the foundation for overall well-being and the pathway to living powerfully with diabetes.

When diet and exercise are not enough to get the cholesterol to an optimal range, adding medications may be beneficial; however, medications do not replace continued lifestyle modifications. I find that a number of people miss the point here and assume that there is no need to continue to adapt healthy lifestyle changes once medications are started just because initial lifestyle modifications through diet and exercise failed.

There are several types of cholesterol-lowering agents. The most common and most studied agents are called the "statins." There are several other classes of medications. Discuss which agent may be optimal for you with your physician.

Whether you are controlling your cholesterol with diet and exercise or pharmaceutical agents, be certain to get regular blood tests to check your fasting lipid profile and chemistries to check your liver function.

Action Steps

Keep a record of your cholesterol. If your cholesterol is outside of the recommended range, have a discussion with your doctor about additional measures that you can take to control it.

Date: _____

Total cholesterol: _____

LDL cholesterol: _____

HDL cholesterol: _____

Triglycerides: _____

Date: _____

Total cholesterol: _____

LDL cholesterol: _____

HDL cholesterol: _____

Triglycerides: _____

M—Microalbumin and Kidney Function

Albumin is a protein found in the blood. Healthy kidneys usually filter it back into circulation. In early kidney damage, microalbumin can be detected in the urine before larger amount of proteins begin to leak into the urine. These small amounts of protein in the urine are detected by a test called the microalbumin test. "Micro" is used to describe the very small amounts of albumin in the urine.

There are some precautions you should take when you are producing a urine sample for a microalbumin test. This is because they may produce what is called a false positive. A false positive can cause you to go through additional tests that are unnecessary and worse still cause you emotional stress which in turn can raise your blood sugars.

So be certain to take the following precautions and also inform your health-care provider about your general state of health:

- Do not touch the edge of the specimen cup with your genital area.
- If you are close to or currently on your menstrual cycle, defer the testing.
- Do not get toilet paper, pubic hair, or any other foreign substance in the specimen cup.
- Do not have the test performed if you have been ill with a fever.
- Persistent high blood sugars can cause a microalbumin leakage in the urine.

If the microalbumin test comes back abnormal, then it needs to be repeated at least two additional times over the next three to six months.

Microalbumin that continues to be detected in the urine is as an early warning sign of early kidney damage. This is a condition called *diabetic nephropathy*. Certain measures can be taken to slow down or prevent further damage to the kidneys. The presence of microalbumin in the urine increases the future risk of developing heart disease.

Unless there are any reasons against this, your doctor will most likely select a medication called an ACE inhibitor. These medications are used to control blood pressure. They are used to treat heart disease, and research studies have also shown them to slow down the progression to full-blown kidney disease in type II diabetes. Be certain to ask your primary care physician about your microalbumin levels and be open to starting an ACE inhibitor.

N—Nutrition

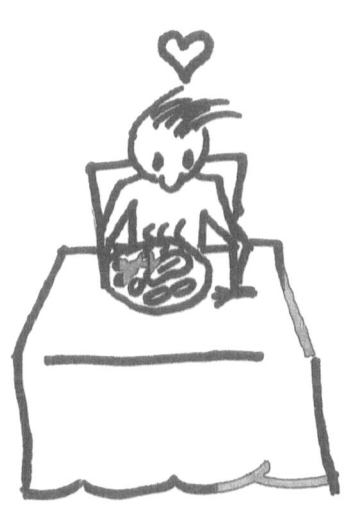 A working knowledge of nutrition is the foundation of living a healthy life. When you have diabetes, it becomes all the more important. Many people get overwhelmed when it comes to nutrition, especially when they hear terms like "carb-counting," "exchanges," "serving sizes," and "recommended daily allowances," among numerous others.

The recommendations outlined in this chapter are obtained from the American Diabetes Association. (For more information, log on to www.diabetes.org.)

My intention is to take the mystery out of nutrition and provide an easy-to-understand guide so that you can begin to apply this into your daily life.

First, I would recommend that you obtain a set of serving cups of different sizes and a food scale.

I shall outline three ways to approach the nutritional aspect of living with diabetes. I encourage you to keep an open mind and experiment with each method. That way you can to decide what fits your lifestyle best.

1. Create Your Plate

Oftentimes when people are first diagnosed with diabetes, they leave the doctor's office overwhelmed. I imagine you felt the same way, mainly because you didn't know where to start. A lot of times, two of the first questions that a patient has are the following: "What am I supposed to eat?" "What kind of diet do I need to be on?"

One of the easiest ways to start out is the "create your plate" method.

I find this to be a much easier method first starting out *before* you begin to learn about the diabetic food pyramid or carb-counting or glycemic index.

Here are the six simple steps to "creating your plate" based on the recommendations of the American Diabetes Association:

- Draw a line down the middle of your dinner plate.
- On one side, draw another line straight down so that your dinner plate is divided into three sections.
- Fill the largest section with nonstarchy vegetables, such as spinach, carrots, lettuce, cauliflower, or broccoli. (You get the idea!)
- In one of the smaller sections, put a starchy food, such as whole grain breads, high-fiber cereal, cooked beans, peas, low-fat crackers, or sweet potatoes. (By now, I trust that you are catching on.)
- In the final section, place your meats or meat substitutes, such a skinless chicken, turkey, lean cuts of beef, or seafood.
- On a small side plate, add a piece of fruit for desert and an eight-ounce serving of a dairy product if you can still tolerate milk, and *voila*, your meal is set!

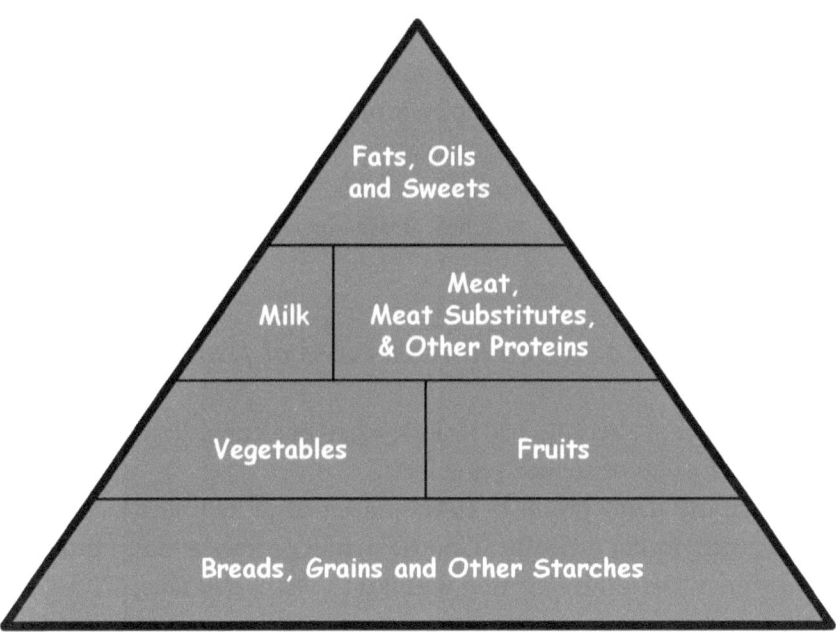

2. The Diabetes Food Pyramid

The diabetes food pyramid divides foods into *six food groups*. The base of the pyramid is composed of the largest group, and it contains grains, beans, and starchy vegetables.

Choose six to eleven servings per day
from Bread, Grains & Starches

An example of a serving size would be one slice of bread, a quarter of a bagel, three quarters of a cup of dry cereal, or a third of a cup of rice or pasta.

Vegetables provide nutrients like vitamins, minerals, and fiber. They are also low in calories. In the diabetic food pyramid, starchy vegetables like potatoes and sweet potatoes are counted in the starch and grain group.

Choose three to five servings a day
from the vegetable group.

The next layer of the pyramid is fruits, which also contain carbohydrates. They also have plenty of vitamins, minerals, fiber, and powerful compounds called antioxidants.

Examples of fruits include blackberries, cantaloupe, strawberries, oranges, apples, bananas, peaches, pears, apricots, and grapes. Choose from a variety of fruits.

Eat between two to four servings of fruits per day.

Examples of a serving size include a half of a cup of raw fruit as well as a half of a cup of cooked vegetables.

Milk and dairy products contain a lot of protein and calcium as well as many other vitamins. Choose nonfat or low-fat dairy products for the great taste and nutrition without the saturated fat.

Choose two to three servings of these per day.

Examples include one cup of nonfat dairy or one cup of nonfat yoghurt.

Meat, Meat substitutes and other proteins

The meat group includes chicken, beef, turkey, fish, and eggs. It also includes tofu, dried beans, cheese, cottage cheese, and peanut butter.

Meat and meat substitutes are great sources of protein as well as many vitamins and minerals.

Lean meats, poultry, and fish are better choices. Try to cut all the visible fat off meat before you cook it. Keep your portion sizes limited to about four to six ounces per day.

Three ounces is about the size of a deck of cards.

Equivalents to 1 oz of meat are as follows: a quarter of a cup of cottage cheese, one egg, one tablespoon of peanut butter or almond butter, and a half of a cup of tofu.

Fats oils and sweets

The smallest size is at the top of the pyramid. These are fats, sweets, and alcohol. You should eat less of these as they have no nutritional value. Divide the number of serving that you eat each day amongst all your meals, including snacks.

3. Carbohydrate Counting

In carbohydrate counting, close attention is paid to the amount of carbohydrates in the diet. Carbohydrates are responsible for the sharp rise in blood sugar levels, especially after you eat. Sharp spikes in blood sugars cause concurrent rises in insulin levels.

There are two types of carbohydrates—*simple carbohydrates and complex carbohydrates.*

Simple carbohydrates are *simple sugars.* They cause the blood sugars to rise rapidly, because they are digested quickly and pass into the blood circulation. Our bodies do not usually need a large amount of sugar at once unless we are involved in intense physical exercise. The excess sugar gets stored in the cells as *glycogen* or fat.

Diabetes develops as a result of either a deficiency in insulin or because the cells become resistant to the actions of insulin (also called insulin resistance). The combined process results in high blood sugar levels.

The body has a limited amount of storage space for these excess sugars. The rest of the sugars that are not broken down into glycogen stores get stored as fat.

Examples of simple carbohydrates are refined sugar, white flour, pastries, candy, sodas, and fruit juices.

On the other hand, complex carbohydrates do not cause a surge in blood sugars. The body has to break down the chains between the carbohydrate molecules before they can be used for fuel. This takes more time and also burns more calories in the process.

Starches and fiber are part of complex carbohydrates, and they are found mostly in plant-based sources.

4. Glycemic Index

The glycemic index measures how much insulin is released to break down the carbohydrates we eat. Here's the rule of thumb:

Foods with a high glycemic index cause more insulin to be released.

Foods with a low glycemic index cause less insulin secretion.

The reference foods white bread or glucose have a GI of one hundred.

The best foods to eat are foods that have a *low* glycemic index (GI).

Foods with a low GI, which is fifty-five or less, tend to raise the blood sugars a lot slower than foods with a high GI.

Examples of such foods include oatmeal (rolled or steel-cut), pasta, stone-ground wheat bread, converted rice, sweet potatoes, corn, yam, beans, legumes, lentils, most fruits, nonstarchy vegetables ,and carrots.

Combining low-GI foods with high-GI foods in one meal would be a good idea. For instance, you may try combining more foods with a low to medium GI, such as dried beans and vegetables, with a smaller portion of foods with a high GI, such as white rice and white breads.

The GI content should only serve as a guide and not be the only way you use to plan your diet. This is because certain foods that have a high nutritional value like oatmeal may also have a high GI. This does not necessarily mean that you need to completely eliminate oatmeal from your diet.

Some Final Guidelines

- Read food labels.
- If you plan on eating a larger portion, keep in mind that you will have to multiply the serving size by the increase in your portion size.
- The recommended range of carbohydrates by the American Diabetes Association is forty-five to sixty grams per meal.
- Be aware of the calorie content of the foods.
- Always be certain to include the other important food groups—proteins and fats.

Restaurant Eating as a Diabetic

Recommendations when you are eating out are commonsense ideas that apply to almost anyone looking to live a healthy lifestyle, and you may want to consider the following tips:

Watch your portion sizes.

Whether eating out or at home, it is important to watch your portion sizes. Most portion sizes in a restaurant are enough for two people. Opt to share with a partner or simply cut the size in half and request a "doggie bag" for lunch the next day.

Make healthy substitutions.

Instead of the French fries, request a baked potato. Opt for low-fat salad dressing instead of regular dressing. Another good option would be to request that the salad dressing is served on the side. Instead of fried foods, opt for broiled or baked items.

Avoid the sides like breads.

By cutting down on the sides like bread, you are able to reduce your amount of calories.

Watch the alcohol intake.

Remember from the diabetic food pyramid that alcohol, which is at the top of the pyramid, is empty calories. If you must drink, opt for light beers, dry wines, or mixed drinks with sugar-free mixes.

Action Plan

Create a shopping list

Review this chapter on nutrition again and write down a list of foods from the different food groups that you would like to incorporate more of into your diet.

Begin to make a conscious practice of reading food labels when you go to the grocery store. See how much of it you can understand. Keep studying food labels a daily practice. Become aware of serving size recommendations.

Keep a food journal

If you got the three subject notebook that I recommended in the journal section, commit to keeping a record of everything that you eat and drink for an entire week.

Include the approximate portion sizes. Also, write a brief memo not more than one or two sentences long. For example, let's say you had an ice cream sundae for dessert. Write in how it made you feel. Or if you found that you craved potato chips, write about how you were feeling when you had the craving. Was it a particularly stressful moment at work? Were you sitting in front of the TV, for instance? Were you bored?

The goal of writing in the food diary is not only to give you an idea of what you are taking into your body in terms of calories but to also allow you to see your existing relationship with food. **It's your relationship with food that you need to work on if you are to live powerfully with diabetes.**

At the end of the week, review your food diary. A lot of people are not aware of how much they actually eat, not to mention the quality of the foods that they eat.

Review your food diary and identify some foods that you can eliminate from your diet or decrease in quantity. Your current goal is to start making small changes. This will result in huge rewards in the future.

For gadget-savvy people, a lot of the smart phones have programs that allow you to keep your food dairy and calculate your total calorie intake.

O—Observe

Observation is a skill that requires that we focus on the present moment, and many times, we do not use this skill fully. It may take a few "hard knocks" to come to the conclusion that certain habits or attitudes need to change as they are having a negative effect on our overall health.

You have to learn to be your own best detective and observe how everything affects you and your overall well-being.

This skill will enable you to be proactive in your approach to your health and your health care. By becoming more proactive, you become more empowered.

Action Plan

Here are some suggested things to observe:

1. Observe and keep a record of how certain foods affect your blood sugar. This will let you make changes, either taking that food out completely if it elevates your blood sugars or putting more of a certain type of food in your diet if you observe that it lowers your blood sugars.
2. Observe whether or not your emotions have an affect your blood sugars.
3. Observe how certain activities may affect your emotions and also your blood sugars.
4. Observe whether there is a relationship between the amount of sleep that you get and your blood sugars.
5. It is very important to be aware of the effects of certain drugs on your body. If you observe any untoward side effects, always communicate your concerns to your physician rather than stopping the medication abruptly.
6. Observe how exercise impacts your blood sugars and make the necessary adjustments. For instance, if your blood sugars tend to drop suddenly after exercise and you observe that, you can make adjustments in your food intake prior to exercise to avert that in the future.

This is just a partial list of things to observe. This is just the beginning of the numerous ways that you can bring more awareness into your daily life by learning the art of observing.

P—Persistence

Being diagnosed with diabetes, can be a life-altering experience. Perhaps you know family members, friends, or associates who may have suffered numerous complications and are now a shell of their old selves.

You could choose that as your reference point, or you could choose a more empowered way to be.

In life, there will be setbacks and challenges along the way. For instance, you may have been able to bring your blood sugars down to the normal range, and then all of the sudden, they seem to be out of control! Life happens, and you are plagued with very significant and stressful events. You may not be able to focus on taking care of your diabetes, or you may encounter another health challenge that overwhelms you.

The fact is life is going to happen. It is how we choose to respond that makes the difference.

Have an attitude of persistence. Continue to press forward no matter what your challenges or setbacks are.

Do not give up on yourself. Do not give in to the negative thoughts that may fill your mind at times, or you will begin to bemoan, "Why me?"

Life is the ultimate journey in self-discovery. I know that may sound so blasé on paper. The truth is you cannot change this diagnosis. Inasmuch as researchers are working hard at finding a cure, the reality is that you are going to have to live with diabetes today!

You can choose to live an empowered life!

Persistence means that you have a choice to determine how your life goes. Welcome each day with an "attitude of gratitude."

Persistence means that you embrace self-responsibility and self-love as the cornerstones of who you are.

It means that you will not stop until you have all your questions answered! You will continue to learn what you need to learn in order to live a more wholesome life.

You will be an active participant in your health care. You will keep yourself informed of the latest developments in the care of people living with diabetes by attending seminars, researching reputable websites online, and reaching out for support when you need it.

Persistence means that you commit to showing up to your life every day.

When you embrace life with persistence, then a stream of possibilities opens up. The Universe will begin to create ways for positive things to happen. It provides you with intuitive insight, which will assist you when you need it.

These are universal and spiritual principles as old as time itself, and they ring true for all of mankind. This is the "law of attraction" in manifestation. What you focus on you attract more of.

So press forward and be persistent!

Action Plan

Practice persistence in small areas first. For instance, notice where you would normally stop and make a conscious effort to press forward.

An example of this may occur if you have committed to walking two miles a day in thirty minutes. You get to thirty minutes and have walked only 1.5 miles. Rather than stopping, "go the extra mile!"

Or perhaps you are challenged by exactly how to calibrate your glucometer. Practice persistence until you figure it out yourself or have someone help you.

Q—Questions

No doubt being diagnosed with any medical condition raises a lot of questions. There will be myriad questions initially, and then as time goes on, you may even have some more questions in between your doctor visits.

The best way to get these questions answered may involve some research on your part or calls to your doctor's office. It is important to be clear about what you are asking.

Write down your questions before your scheduled appointments with your doctors.

For instance, be clear about the target sugars that your doctor has set for you. If you are not certain about how to approach a certain aspect of your care, then place a call to your doctor's office and get immediate clarification.

Never assume anything when it comes to your care. Don't be afraid to ask questions.

You may also want to research answers to your questions using resources, such as the Internet or reading materials like this book.

Be certain that you are using reputable resources online, because there are a lot of sites online that may give misleading information. When you are researching online, be sure to review information about the same topic from several reputable sites.

If your physician allows e-mail correspondence, this may also be another way to get questions answered. Be certain to check with your physician whether or not this is a method of communication that is supported by their office, for measures have to be in place to protect confidential patient information.

Action Plan

A day or two before your scheduled appointment with your doctor, take time to write out a list of questions.

R—Referrals

Referrals are a very important component of your diabetes care. There are a number of specialists that you will need to see on a routine or as-needed basis. Below is a list of the more common referrals for most people with diabetes:

Endocrinologist

Your primary care provider may decide to refer you to a specialist in diabetes and other diseases of the glands. This specialist is called an endocrinologist. It may be necessary if your sugars continue to remain out of control and require a more complicated regimen to achieve good sugar control.

Remember that the ultimate goal is to get your sugars well controlled.

Ophthalmologist

An ophthalmologist is a physician who specializes in the management and treatment of eye diseases. Diabetes is a leading cause of blindness worldwide, and it is important to detect early changes in the eyes in order to avoid future complications. It is important to see an ophthalmologist every year.

At times, you may also need to be referred to another ophthalmology specialist called a *retinal specialist*. This is especially important if there is any evidence of bleeding in the back of the eye as this can lead to blindness of not treated promptly. Retinal laser surgery can help stop the small blood vessels from bleeding.

Podiatrist

A podiatrist is a foot specialist and serves as a very important aspect of preventive care. It is even more important to seek the regular care of a podiatrist if your toenails are overgrown or you have foot deformities. A podiatrist may also recommend special orthotics or shoes if you have foot deformities.

Dentist

Do not neglect to see your dentist every six months. There is a strong association between gum disease and heart disease.

Cardiologist

This is a specialist in heart disease and works closely with your primary care doctor. If you have heart disease, then you may need to see a cardiologist. At times, it may be necessary to see a cardiologist as part of a preventive program. For instance, you may visit one to get a stress test before you start an exercise program.

Nephrologist

Nephrologists are medical doctors that specialize in kidney diseases. There is a misconception amongst diabetics that once they are referred to a kidney specialist, this means that they are going to start dialysis. This is not always the case. There are several stages of kidney disease. Most of the time, if problems with your kidneys are caught early, then working with a kidney specialist may help prevent the progression to full-blown kidney disease.

Action Plan

Keep up with referrals to specialists that your primary care physician sends you to. Mark the dates on your calendar so that you do not forget them.

S—Supplements

Many people with diabetes attempt to control their blood sugars naturally without the use of pharmaceutical medications. The overall goal should be to keep blood sugars within a safe range. This will help reduce the complications that are associated with poorly controlled blood sugars.

It is very important, however, to work closely with your physician if you consider using complementary and alternative medicine (also known as CAM). If you have already been started on prescription medications, this should not replace conventional medicine.

If you choose to use CAM, be certain that your doctor is conversant with the different supplements that you are using.

The following is a summary of studied CAM therapies that may be of benefit in the management of diabetes. During my clinical practice, I made recommendations that incorporated some of these therapies. However, I in no way endorse this as the exclusive way to treat diabetes.

ALPHA LIPOIC ACID (ALA)

Also known as lipoic acid or thioctic acid, this is an antioxidant. Antioxidants help protect the cells from damage by free radicals. ALA is unique in the way that it works. Compared to other antioxidants that may work in water, such as Vitamin C, fats, and Vitamin E, ALA works both ways. Levels of alpha lipoic acid begin to decline with age. Because ALA may lower the blood sugars drastically, it is important to monitor blood sugars closely when on this supplement.

OMEGA-3 FATTY ACIDS

These are fats that are unsaturated. They are commonly called fish oils. They are much harder to come by in our diets. They are present in small concentrations in leafy vegetables, seeds, nuts, flax seed, and hemp. Omega-3 fatty acids are more commonly found in fish like the wild Alaskan salmon, sardine, tuna, and mackerel.

Studies have shown that omega-3 fatty acids lower triglycerides; however, they do not affect the sugar control or total cholesterol. Triglyceride levels are usually elevated in diabetics, and they have been found to increase the risk for heart disease. Omega-3 fatty acid supplements appear to be safe in low to moderate doses.

Because of safety concerns about some species of fish contaminated by mercury and pesticides and PCB, I strongly recommend that you use only supplements that have been certified by the NNFA (National Nutritional Foods Association) as GMP certified.

Omega-3 fatty acids may also increase your risk of bleeding during surgery.

CHROMIUM

Chromium is a trace mineral. Trace minerals are only required in very small amounts in the body. Chromium is found in small amounts in meat, whole grain products, and some fruits and vegetables. Some people take chromium supplements in an attempt to control blood sugars; however, studies have shown mixed benefits. Some studies have shown a benefit, and others did not. At low doses, it may be of benefit; however, as with any other supplements, it may lower blood sugars to dangerous levels. **In high doses, chromium can lead to kidney problems.**

POLPYPHENOLS

These are antioxidants that are found in tea and also dark chocolate. They may have positive effects on the circulation and blood pressure. A polyphenol called *EGCG* in green tea has been found to protect against heart disease. Studies performed by the National Center for Complementary and Alternative Medicine have not confirmed this in diabetics. However, there were no bad side effects noted in the study. Overall, green tea in moderate amounts has been found to be safe in adults.

CINNAMON

Cinnamon has also been researched as possibly lowering blood sugar levels. Cinnamon may have an *insulin-like effect.*

The most cited scientific study on the effects of cinnamon and diabetes was published in the *Journal of Diabetes Care* in 2003. Individuals in the cinnamon group were noted to have reductions in their glucose by up to 29 percent, and this was found to last up to forty days after they had stopped taking cinnamon. They also found a change in the cholesterol and the triglyceride levels, which was an additional benefit. The downside is that this effect was not replicated in another study carried out in Germany. There are also some concerns that some forms of cinnamon may contain a compound called coumarin, which is a blood thinner. So inasmuch as cinnamon has gotten a lot of attention about "sugar-busting benefits," the jury is still out there!

Other noteworthy supplements that have been studied for diabetes-related benefits are as follows:

- Garlic may lower blood glucose. Benefits have not been consistent.
- Magnesium as a supplement for control of blood sugars received mixed results. Researchers did find that a diet rich in magnesium lowered the risk of developing diabetes. Magnesium is found in whole grain and vegetables such as spinach, plantains, black beans, and tofu. In addition, it is also found in fish, such as rockfish, scallops, and halibut.

- There have been conflicting findings about coenzyme Q10 in sugar control.
- There are ongoing studies on the benefits of ginseng and another trace mineral called vanadium and their effects on glucose control.
- Finally, other botanicals like bitter melon, prickly pear cactus, gurmar, coccinia indica, aloe vera, and fenugreek have been tried as well.

According to the National Institute for Complementary and Alternative Medicine, there are no conclusive studies documenting any of these as beneficial.

Here are some precautions to take if you are diabetic and considering adding a supplement to your regimen:

- If you are pregnant or planning to get pregnant, do not use a dietary supplement.
- Discuss all supplements that you are taking with your doctor so that he or she can get a full picture of all the medications you are taking.
- Do not replace your prescription medications with alternative medicines

Action Plan

For more information about current CAM therapies, I recommend that you log on to the National Complementary and Alternative Therapy website.

T—Treat Promptly

Frequently, our human nature makes us second guess or procrastinate perhaps because we may fear that we are reading too much into our symptoms or we may not have a clear understanding about them. We do not want to unnecessarily alarm family or friends or even ourselves!

However, it is important to seek medical attention immediately if you experience any new symptoms or develop any new signs.

The age old adage "an ounce of prevention is worth a pound of cure" rings true all around.

I would rather have a diabetic see me for a symptom that they were not sure about than label it "irrelevant" only to find out months later that they had a more serious complication.

- Examples abound about common symptoms that may become more serious issues. For instance, athlete's foot between the toes may become a serious bacterial infection with an underlying infection of the bone (osteomyelitis). This could lead to very serious side effects or even the amputation of a limb.
- Persistent heartburn could indicate heart disease.
- Blurry vision could mean bleeding in the back of the eye.

Symptoms can only be treated promptly when you observe and communicate your concerns to your physician in a timely manner.

When in doubt ask, ask, and ask again. Become a walking question mark!

U—Utilize a Support System

When living with diabetes, it is important to utilize the available support systems within your health-care network but also develop a strong social support system of your own.

A diabetic support system may consist of several ancillary staff, including your doctor(s).

These may include a diabetic educator, a nutritionist, a registered nurse or nurse practitioner, and specialists. (See the section on referrals.) Depending on your insurance, you may even have access to a personal trainer or an exercise physiologist.

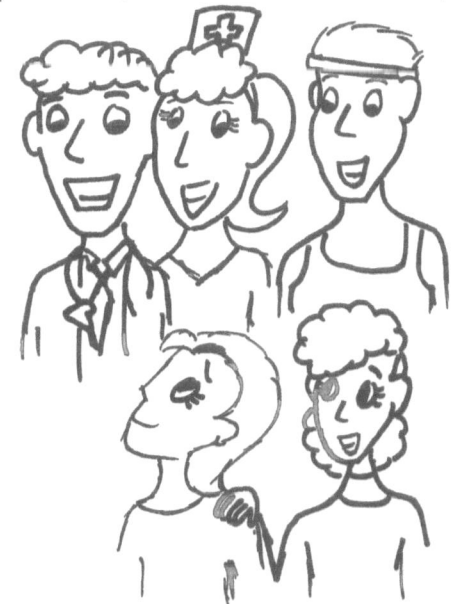

These specialists are all very important parts of the team that you will use to help you maintain a healthy life. Get to know the team members well, and do not hesitate to ask your physician for referrals to different members of the support team.

For instance, if after you have read the chapter on nutrition, you are still uncertain about how to eat healthy and in a way that will help control your blood sugars, then by all means see a nutritionist.

You may have just been started on insulin and want to learn how to inject it properly. Then you may need to enlist the services of a nurse educator and a diabetes educator.

You may want to hire a personal trainer or an exercise physiologist, especially if this is one of the benefits that your employer offers.

Perhaps you want to learn how you may design a ***customized wellness plan*** that takes into account every aspect of your life. This plan is designed with goals you want to reach. This is where a ***wellness coach like myself***, would work with you. Together we create a partnership where you are committed to produce the results that you want for your life. I have found this to produce lasting transformations, well beyond what I experienced as a physician. And this is why I am committed to the bringing an awareness of the powerful benefits that exist for improving health through coaching.

Another important part of your team is the support team you assemble yourself. This may include family members, friends, or colleagues.

The support structure that you set up must be a positive influence in your life. At times, things may get a little overwhelming, and your sugars may begin to rise. You may feel like giving up on yourself, but if you have a strong support system, your support team that will encourage you.

V—Vacation

Vacations and recreation are an important part of rest, rejuvenation, and relaxation.

Too often we tend to get caught up in the day-to-day grind of existence.

At times, the toll of the diagnosis of a chronic illness may temporarily rob us of our enjoyment of life. It may also place stress on family, particularly our intimate relationships.

Vacations are a valuable time to reconnect with ourselves and those we love. They serve as times to evaluate what matters most in our lives.

When you are planning a vacation, allow yourself to dream again. By dreaming, you are using the right side of the brain, which allow us to increase our innate creativity.

Think of the things that you enjoy to doing for "recreation."

Practical Tips for Travel

There are, however, certain practical issues to consider when you are taking a vacation away from home.

If you require insulin, be sure to carry your insulin pens as part of your carry-on baggage. For the most part, you may not need to place this on ice, as most of the insulin today may be kept at room temperature for up to thirty days once the vial or pen is opened. Avoid extreme temperature fluctuations.

Ensure that you obtain refills of all your medications, including your testing supplies, before you leave, especially if you are planning to travel out of the country.

It is also a good idea to have some form of identification showing that you are a diabetic and/or require insulin.

Action Plan

Think about what your dream vacation might be like. Picture the destination, the people you would be with, and the activities that you would engage in while there. Create a vivid picture in your mind's eye. Imagine the sounds, and if possible, imagine the smells and what you'd wear. Close your eyes and relax into that dream destination.

How does this make you feel?

Make a commitment to vacation at least once a year or take mini-vacations like four-day weekends several times a year.

For some ideas on vacation destinations or to book an upcoming vacation, you can log onto my online travel website at www.wellcarevacations.com.

W—Well-Being and Wellness

A lot of times when you are dealing with chronic medical problems like diabetes, it is not uncommon that this overshadows other aspects of your health.

Be sure to get annual wellness checks. Try to make this annual visit separate from your routine diabetes care so that full attention can be directed to your wellness.

Examples of things to get done at an annual wellness check include the following:

- Ensure that you are current with all your immunizations.
- For women, get annual pelvic examinations and Pap smears.
- A woman over the age of forty years old should get annual breast examinations from her physician and annual mammograms.
- If you are an African American male over the age of forty years, you should get an annual prostate check and a PSA.
- People over the age of fifty years should get a screening colon test called a colonoscopy.
- Everyone should get several blood tests, including complete blood counts (CBCs), thyroid screens (TSHs), and complete blood chemistries.

- If you have not already had your blood tests done as part of your diabetes care, then this can be combined into the wellness panel.

The annual wellness checkup should be used as an opportunity to discuss other prevention and wellness issues with your health-care provider. The focus should be on strategies to increase your level of wellness.

Just because you have been diagnosed with a chronic illness like diabetes does not mean that you cannot aspire to live a healthy lifestyle. In fact, this should be your goal at all times.

Wellness

We are exposed to a lot of information on health and well-being. In order to create a wellness lifestyle, it is important to take action with the knowledge that we acquire. Too often, our system of health care tends to focus on the sickness model. In this model, a patient sees a doctor when something is wrong and remains in a somewhat passive role in that interaction. The patient may not ask too many questions about why or how they got sick, and is there just demanding to be made well. Naturally this kind of interaction encourages unrealistic expectations on the part of the patient and at times the family members who usually only become involved when major illness strikes.

Health and wellness are not static states. I like to say that **"Healthcare is equal to wealth care."** Without your health and well-being, it is literally impossible to be fully functional in other areas of your life.

Think about how chronic illnesses like diabetes can actually serve as a springboard for your personal growth. It could mean giving good care to your physical body, feeding your mind with positive thoughts, creating a support system that empowers you, and being concerned about your spiritual and psychological well-being.

When I coach my clients, a lot of my work centers on creating an empowered relationship to their health and well-being. This is irrespective of whether they are dealing with any chronic illness.

e**X**cellence

Strive for excellence in all that you do. This is a lesson for all of life, not just for living with diabetes.

If you knew you could not fail, what would be possible for you?

There are many celebrities who have diabetes and have gone on to live very productive lives that continue to make an impact on those around them.

Think of ways that you can create a positive awareness of what it takes to live a healthy lifestyle as a diabetic. It may be something as simple as speaking words of encouragement to someone who has just been recently diagnosed with diabetes and is bewildered and has no idea how this is going to impact his or her life. Give him or her a copy of this manual. Become a walking ambassador of what it means to live with diabetes.

I used to reward all my diabetic patients with a pin that stated they had achieved an A1C of less than 7 percent. I am proud to say that the majority have been able to maintain their A1C at less than 7 percent because they have a vested interest. I demand the pin back if their A1C goes higher than 7 percent for two consecutive quarters! These patients are walking ambassadors who wear that pin with pride, and they also strive to live in excellence in order to keep the words true—A1C less than 7 percent.

Y—Yes, You Can!

At the end of the day, it's all about *you*. What matters most to you? You are the most important person in your arena. How you deal with yourself and your diagnosis determines how well you will live life overall.

I have covered several aspects related to your mindset—acceptance, belief, persistence, observation, and questioning. These aspects all help you become more empowered as you embrace living well with diabetes.

You have a choice, and I hope that by the time you have reached this chapter, you are your best ally. I hope that you believe enough in your inner ability to move forward. If so, then my mission for this book has been fulfilled.

Z—Zero in with Zest!

The dictionary definition of zest is "spirited enjoyment." Create enthusiasm in your daily life. I couldn't help ending this book with a play on words, one that I hope will bring a smile to your lips.

Diabetes is a chronic medical condition, but it does not have to translate to a death sentence.

There are countless people around the globe who live healthy and productive lives with diabetes. They each go about their daily lives with a zest for living, self-acceptance, self-discovery, willingness to change, a strong belief in their abilities, and a higher force.

Living life with zest means focusing on the positive things and what you have control over. It is being open to life's possibilities.

Be playful, and enjoy life. You have only one chance to live in this body. There is no space for regrets or "what ifs." Zero in with zest!

Appendix

The appendix contains materials that I compiled as a resource for my patients when I was working in an office-based practice. I offer this as a guide only.

Please consult your health-care provider about your medical condition before you implement the recommendations contained herein.

Instructions for
Checking Blood Sugars:

CHECK YOUR BLOOD SUGAR FIRST THING IN THE MORNING BEFORE YOU EAT. THE NORMAL LEVEL SHOULD BE BETWEEN *80–120 MG/DL*.

IF YOUR BLOOD SUGARS ARE HIGHER THAN 140 MG/DL OR LESS THAN 60 MG/DL, THEN PLEASE INFORM YOUR PRIMARY DOCTOR.

ALSO CHECK YOUR SUGARS *TWO HOURS* AFTER YOU EAT. CHOOSE ANY MEAL OF YOUR CHOICE. YOUR BLOOD SUGARS SHOULD BE *LESS THAN 140 MG/DL*.

THERE IS A SIMPLE WAY YOU MAY USE TO CHECK YOUR SUGARS. ALTERNATE CHECKING YOUR FASTING SUGARS AND YOUR SUGARS AFTER YOU EAT AS FOLLOWS: DIVIDE THE MONTH INTO ODD NUMBERERED DAYS AND EVEN NUMBERED DAYS. ON THE ODD NUMBERED DAYS, CHECK YOUR SUGARS FIRST THING IN THE MORNING, AND ON EVEN NUMBERED DAYS OF THE MONTH, CHECK YOUR SUGARS TWO HOURS AFTER YOUR MEAL.

IF YOU ARE WORKING A SCHEDULE WHERE IT IS NOT CONVENIENT TO CHECK YOUR SUGARS DURING THE WEEK, THEN DO TWO-HOUR SUGAR CHECKS DURING THE WEEKEND, STARTING FRIDAY EVENING. (NOTE THAT YOU DO NOT HAVE TO CHECK YOUR SUGARS FIRST THING IN THE MORNING OR OVER THE WEEKEND IF YOU CHOOSE THIS REGIMEN, BUT YOU CAN. IT JUST GIVES YOUR DOCTOR MORE READINGS TO REVIEW.)

HERE ARE SOME THINGS YOU SHOULD BRING TO YOUR NEXT DOCTOR'S VISIT:

PLEASE WRITE DOWN YOUR SUGARS IN YOUR LOG BOOK AND BRING IT TO YOUR DOCTOR'S APPOINTMENT. ALSO BRING IN YOUR GLUCOSE METER.

IF YOU HAVE ANY QUESTIONS, PLEASE DO NOT HESITATE TO CONTACT YOUR DOCTOR.

Healthy Nutrition and Weight Management Personalized Worksheet

Below is a worksheet that I give to my patients as part of their annual health maintenance. Please check with your primary care physician about these recommendations before you implement them in your lifestyle.

1) Dietary Supplements

Consider a good multivitamin supplement that contains at least 400 micrograms of folic acid and at least 600 IU of Vitamin D. They should not contain any iron and preformed Vitamin A. Always ensure that the supplement is independently certified by GMP or NNFA.

Women should also take supplemental calcium, preferably citrate. Daily needs range between 1,200–1,500 mg per day for most postmenopausal women without a diagnosis of osteoporosis.

For osteoporosis or osteopenia, I recommend 2,000 mg of calcium as follows: Take two tablets twice a day with meals. Your doctor may also recommend the addition of another agent to treat the osteoporosis.

Omega-3 fish oils may help, and you should start at one or two grams per day. Look for molecularly distilled products that are certified and free of mercury and other heavy metal contents.

Speak with your doctor about low-dose aspirin therapy.

If you have joint pains or have been diagnosed with arthritis, you may want to use turmeric and ginger in your diet or supplements.

(Consider this good recipe for ginger tea. Grate a ginger root and steep it in hot water until it cools down. Then you can serve your tea. Sweeten with Stevia or raw brown sugar to taste.)

Consider sixty to a hundred milligrams of Co-Q with the largest meal. You may require a higher dosage if you are on cholesterol-lowering statin agents.

If you have been diagnosed with *metabolic syndrome*, consider taking a hundred to four hundred milligrams of alpha-lipoic acid per day.

If you have hypertension, I recommend calcium-magnesium supplementation. Try to obtain a supplement with calcium citrate, or else you may want to get separate components as follows: four hundred milligrams of magnesium oxide taken twice daily and calcium citrate as I have described above.

2) Nutrition

Choose fruits and vegetables from all parts of the color spectrum. For instance, you could pick cantaloupe, honey dew melon, tomatoes, broccoli, and leafy vegetables like kale, collard greens, and spinach.

Reduce the consumption of foods with a high glycemic index. They will increase the release of insulin, and they are also prone to increase hot flashes in postmenopausal women.

Combine foods with a high glycemic index with foods that have a low glycemic index.

For a list of foods and their glycemic index, please visit www. mendosa.com/gilists.htm.

Fatty fish are a great source of fiber and also plant derived Omega-3. Blend seeds and spread them on dishes, soups, beverages, salads, bowls of cereal—you name it! Get creative with ways to increase your intake of good nutrition.

Increase the intake of soy. Try different forms, such as soy milk, tofu, and tempeh.

Reduce the consumption of meats, especially red meats, to about six ounces per serving. Chicken is a better source. Reduce frying foods, and broil or bake more. If you do fry foods, do not overheat your oils, because this will change the composition of the oils. If possible, try to eliminate meat completely from your diet. Try doing this for thirty days and see how you feel.

Use Stevia as a natural sweetener. It does not contain any calories and does not affect the glycemic index.

3) Fiber

Increase the amount of fiber in your diet to preferably thirty-five to forty grams per day. Good sources fiber include oat bran cereal (4–5 grams per serving), kashi cereal (8 grams per serving), blue berries (40 grams per serving), and steel-cut oats (*not* instant oatmeal). (Soak your oats overnight, because they will be easier to cook the next morning.) Remember that soy is also a good source of fiber!

4) Increased Physical Activity

Purchase a pedometer from your local sports store. Be sure to calibrate this using the instructions that are enclosed with it.

Your goal is to start increasing your physical activity each day by aiming for ten thousand steps.

Start simply. Wear your pedometer all day long, and at the end of the day, see how many steps you have walked. Aim to increase your steps each day by five hundred steps until you reach your goal of ten thousand steps. You'll find that you will need to dedicate at least thirty minutes of exercise to walking each day to reach your goal of ten thousand steps.

And what do you do once you reach your goal of ten thousand steps? Then set another goal of fifteen thousand steps per day. *You can do it!*

Remember to wear good sneakers while you are walking and change your sneakers after every five hundred miles!

5) Practice Deep Breathing Exercises Several Times a Day

Deep breathing helps with the reduction of stress. Practice this exercise several times a day: Become conscious of your breath. Notice your breathing as you inhale and exhale normally. Gradually increase the depth of your inhalation to expand the bottom of your lungs, and without holding your breath, exhale out as much as you can. Continue to do this for a total of five repetitions. If you feel dizzy at any point, then decrease the depth of your breathing. As you become more accustomed to deep breathing, increase your depth and repetitions.

You may also want to do this exercise at bedtime while you are lying down and you are unable to "switch off" the intruding thoughts of the day.

Resource List

American Diabetes Association
1701 North Beauregard Street
Alexandria, VA 22311
(800) 342-2383
www.diabetes.org

American Association of Diabetes Educators (AADE)
200 W. Madison, Suite 800
Chicago, IL 60606
800-338-3633 www.aadenet.org

National Kidney Foundation,
30 East 33rd Street
New York, NY 10016
800-622-9010
www.kidney.org

The Heart of Diabetes (American Heart Association)
7272 Greenville Avenue
Dallas, TX 75231
800-AHA-USA1
www.s2mw.com/heartofdiabetes/index.html

American Dietetic Association
120 S. Riverdale Plaza, Suite 2000
Chicago, IL 60606-6995
800-877-1600
www.eatright.org

BD Medical—Diabetes Care1 Becton Drive
Franklin Lakes, NJ 07417-1880
Phone: 888-232-2737
www.bddiabetes.com/us

SAY YES TO YOUR WELL-BEING!

Thank you for purchasing this book. Great news! Your journey is just beginning and it is my mission to continue to support you to live a powerful life with diabetes.

So join me online at my interactive blog site created just for you www. PowerfulLivingDiabetes.com

The purpose of this blog is to engage you my reader in a conversation about living powerfully with type II diabetes.

How do you know this may be what you have been looking for?

You would like to decode what your doctor really means to tell you about type II diabetes.

You want to learn about type II diabetes in language that is easy to understand.

You do not what to be a STATISTIC of the complications associated with poorly controlled diabetes.

You are looking for a tool that will allow you to better partner with your physician to enhance your wellbeing.

You would like learning how like my former patients you too can create an unstoppable belief that motivates you to create a powerful life.

Log on right now to www.PowerfulLivingDiabetes.com and Join the Diabetes Buzz!!

To your Health and Wellbeing

Dr Eno

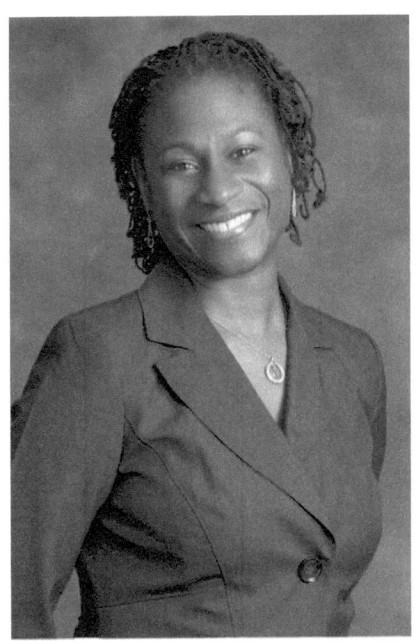

Born in London and raised in Nigeria, Dr. Eno Nsima-Obot is a board certified physician in Internal Medicine, with over 20 years of experience in the health & wellness industry. She graduated from medical school in 1987 with awards in Obstetrics & Gynecology and Clinical Pharmacology. She was also the recipient for the quarterly award for compassion when she worked at a large multi-specialty medical group.

She is an internationally sought after speaker and life coach and has appeared on TV and radio.

As a physician, her philosophy of practice is to provide her patients with enough information to make powerful health choices.

This motivated her to write this book which is designed to empower individuals living with Type II Diabetes. The book is a byproduct of the success she experienced whilst in clinical practice where she found that by providing her patients with easy to understand information on Diabetes, they were motivated to better control their blood sugars by adapting healthier life styles and ways of being.

Dr Eno currently resides in the greater Chicago land area with her husband, teenage daughter and adoring West Highland Terrier (Russell)

For more information about Dr Eno including her current coaching programs, seminars and wellness retreats log onto www.askdoctoreno.com

'Our Chief want in life is somebody who will make us do what we can'

—Ralph Waldo Emerson

www.ingramcontent.com/pod-product-compliance
Lightning Source LLC
Chambersburg PA
CBHW022009170526
45157CB00003B/1201